2 MINUTE MEDICINE™

concise. curated. evi

THE CLASSICS SE ™

2 MINUTE MEDICINE'S THE CLASSICS IN RADIOLOGY™

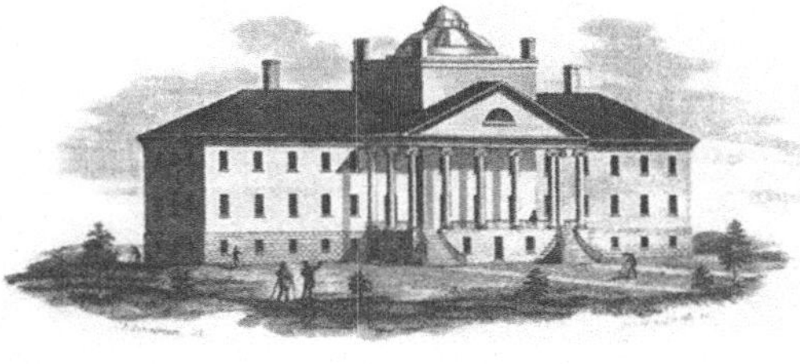

FIRST EDITION

MARC D. SUCCI, MD
Massachusetts General Hospital Department of Radiology
Harvard Medical School

RAVI V. GOTTUMUKKALA, MD
Massachusetts General Hospital Department of Radiology
Harvard Medical School

2 Minute Medicine™

Physician Press™

2 Minute Medicine, Inc.
PO Box 140373
Boston, MA 02114
USA

2 MINUTE MEDICINE'S THE CLASSICS IN RADIOLOGY

ISBN-13: 978-0-9963042-8-3

Library of Congress Cataloging-in-Publication Data

Names: Succi, Marc D., author | Gottumukkala, Ravi V., author
Title: 2 Minute Medicine's The Classics in Radiology / [authored by] Marc D. Succi, Ravi V. Gottumukkala
Other titles: The classics in radiology (Succi)
Description: Summaries of Clinically Relevant & Recent Landmark Studies | Boston, MA: 2 Minute Medicine, [2018] | Includes bibliographical references and index.
Identifiers: LCCN 2018914582 | ISBN 9780996304283 (alk. paper)
Subjects: LCSH: Diagnosis, Radioscopic. | Diagnostic Imaging. | Magnetic resonance imaging. | Oncology. | Clinical trials.
Classification: LCC RC78.S69 | NLM WN 180 | DDC 616.07/57-dc23

International Standard Book Number: 978-0-9963042-8-3
Project Manager: Marc Succi
Content Strategist: Marc Succi, Ravi Gottumukkala
Cover Art: The Anatomy Lesson of Dr. Nicolaes Tulp; 1632, Rembrandt Harmenszoon van Rijn.

2 Minute Medicine™
Physician Press™
2 Minute Medicine, Inc.
PO Box 140373
Boston, MA 02114
USA

About | 2 Minute Medicine creates and curates expert, original, and peer-reviewed medical content. With thousands of published medical reports syndicated worldwide and updated daily on www.2minutemedicine.com, 2 Minute Medicine is the definitive source for curated, updated and authoritative medical news. 2 Minute Medicine conducts academic studies in medical education and has presented its data, by invitation, at numerous international peer-reviewed conferences.

For bulk orders and licenses of 2 Minute Medicine services and products, see www.2minutemedicine.com/license-content.

THE CLASSICS SERIES™

Explore other books in 2 Minute Medicine's *The Classics Series™*

2 Minute Medicine's The Classics in Medicine
Summaries of the Landmark Trials, 1st Edition (2015)
Marc D. Succi, Leah H. Carr, Andrew Cheung

2 Minute Medicine's The Classics in Medicine
Summaries of the Landmark Trials, 2nd Edition (2019)
Marc D. Succi, Leah H. Carr, Andrew Cheung

Available on Amazon, iTunes, Barnes & Noble, and at bookstores worldwide

"In general, we look for a new law by the following process. First, we guess it. Then we compute the consequences of the guess to see what would be implied if this law that we guessed is right. Then we compare the result of the computation to nature, with experiment or experience, compare it directly with observation, to see if it works. If it disagrees with experiment, it's wrong.

In that simple statement is the key to science.

It doesn't make any difference how beautiful your guess is. It doesn't make any difference how smart you are, who made the guess, or what his name is.

If it disagrees with experiment it's wrong. That's all there is to it."

-Richard P. Feynman, PhD

Winner of the Nobel Prize in Physics (1965)

This page left intentionally blank.

CONTENTS

This page left intentionally blank.

FOREWORD

Radiology is a relatively young specialty. The first scientific discoveries in the field were published very shortly after Roentgen's discovery of the x-ray in 1895. Early publications were merely descriptive in nature, carefully detailing imaging findings in multiple disease states. As technological advances occurred with the advent of computed tomography and magnetic resonance imaging, comparative studies of the efficacy of different imaging modalities followed. The past few decades have witnessed not only an explosion of knowledge in the field of radiology but a much more rigorous approach to research based on experimental studies and clinical trials. The transition from printed to digital media and the birth of the internet age have contributed to an exponential increase in the imaging literature. Unfortunately, it has also lead to an increase in low quality and non-peer reviewed evidence.

Part of my responsibility as an educator and program director for many years has been to instill a nuanced understanding of the literature in our trainees in order to prepare them to excel in both patient care and in medical research. Evidence based medicine expressed in trials and consensus statements such as the Fleischner guidelines provide the underpinning for our clinical practice in radiology. The value of *2 Minute Medicine's The Classics in Radiology*™ lies in a thoughtful curation and efficient organization of individual classic studies in radiology. It comprises literature that every resident trainee and radiologist should know in order to excel in the interpretation of images, the performance of interventional procedures, and ultimately the exemplary care of patients. It includes individual studies, trials, consensus statements, as well as aggregated meta-analyses and systemic reviews. The authors, in collaboration with leading radiologists, provide thoughtful summaries of these publications, allowing the learner to master the foundational literature which supports and underlies both appropriateness criteria and practice guidelines.

Sincerely,

Theresa C. McLoud, MD
Associate Radiologist in Chief
Program Director, Massachusetts General Hospital Radiology Residency
Professor of Radiology, Harvard Medical School
Director of Education
Thoracic Imaging Division, Massachusetts General Hospital

This page left intentionally blank.

PREFACE

To my parents and family, thank-you for your unwavering support in my medical education and extra-curricular pursuits. To Dr. Robert Novelline, thank-you for demonstrating the true meaning of an exemplary medical educator and encouraging my pursuit of radiology. To Dr. Alexander Ball, your masterful teaching of human anatomy has been indispensable in clinical practice.

-Marc D. Succi, MD

To my parents and brother Rajesh, thank you for your boundless love and support. To my dearest friends Vivek and Vidit, thank you for constantly inspiring me to try and match your brilliance and for an endless supply of laughs. To Dr. Sanjeev Bhalla, thank you for providing me with the vision of what it means to embody the consummate diagnostic radiologist.

-Ravi V. Gottumukkala, MD

The authors would like to express a sincere appreciation for the academic culture in the Department of Radiology at the Massachusetts General Hospital. It is only through collaboration and academic camaraderie that ventures such as this book are possible. We have received support from countless individuals within the Department of Radiology, from feedback on this book content to general encouragement.

The authors also extend a personal thanks to several individuals in the Department of Radiology administration, including Dr. James A. Brink, Dr. Theresa C. McLoud, Dr. Michael S. Gee, Dr. Raul N. Uppot, Jae Lee, Melanie Miller, and Noemi Chavez. Your encouragement and support in the department, residency program, and beyond is invaluable.

Over the past 30 years, the transition from print to digital media has contributed to an exponential increase in imaging literature. This information overload is revolutionizing the implementation of evidence-based medicine in radiology. Robust trials and consensus statements such as the Fleischner Society Guidelines, ROMICAT, MR-CLEAN, LUNG-RADS, PI-RADS, as well as select breaking trials such as the DAWN, DEFUSE 3, EXTEND-IA TNK and many more underlie our daily decisions in clinical practice. With a plethora of landmark cases occupying isolated corners of both print and digital publications, there exists a tangible need to collect, curate, and summarize these studies in one place for the benefit of all health professionals.

In response, 2 Minute Medicine presents a curated collection of authoritative and physician-written summaries of the most influential, practice-changing landmark studies in radiology: 2 Minute Medicine's The Classics in Radiology™. Every imaging physician, health professional, and trainee should have a working knowledge of these studies to both understand and make daily evidence-based clinical decisions. With contributions from renowned medical faculty and practicing physicians at top institutions, 2 Minute Medicine's The Classics in Radiology is an indispensable tool for the practicing general radiologist or trainee.

Sections in this text are framed on four key areas of knowledge for the reader:

> I. Foundational Literature - Fleischner, ROMICAT, NEXUS, PIOPED, etc.
> II. Screening Literature - BI-RADS, PI-RADS, LI-RADS, LUNG-RADS, etc.
> III. Interventional Literature – DAWN, DEFUSE, EXTEND-IA TNK, RAPTURE, ICTUS, EVAR, RIVAL, etc.
> IV. Interface Literature - RECIST 1.1, NASCET, NINDS, Harvey-Bradshaw Index, Milan Criteria, etc.

The advanced radiologist may choose to focus on sections II-IV, but we believe all sections are critical to daily practice. Specifically, *IV. Interface Literature* includes study summaries that radiologist often must have a working knowledge of to effectively consult with other specialties, such as oncology, surgery, etc. This section includes notable studies such as RECIST 1.1, INVEST, NASCEST, ECASS, NINDS, and many more. We hope advanced radiologists will find this section useful.

The text summaries themselves are organized according to 2 Minute Medicine's signature tiered writing style. Features include key points, a quick "Study Rundown", and an "In-Depth" section for examining key details that one may wish to refer to when citing the study. As always, every medical summary cites the original study. In the e-book edition, this takes the form of a direct web link within the summary to the specific trial on the publishing journal's website in addition to a comprehensive bibliography at the end of the book. In the paperback version, references are cited at the end of each study summary as well as in a comprehensive bibliography at the end of the book.

This book is dedicated to the researchers who create the knowledge, the clinicians that practice it, the teachers who spread it, and the students that learn from it.

Sincerely,

Marc D. Succi, MD & Ravi V. Gottumukkala, MD

Effectively Using this Book

A note on the subspecialties included:

The rise of subspecialization within radiology has been a core component of modern imaging. However, the reality is that disease does not respect artificial boundaries. Thus, many of these study summaries could fit under multiple subspecialties. To prioritize readability, the editors organized studies according to body part, each section beginning with thoracic imaging. Typically, though not always, summaries are sorted in ascending order by date, though priority is given to more influential trials. For example, the recent landmark trials in neurointerventional radiology, such as DAWN, DEFUSE, and EXTEND-IA, are given priority placement earlier in "III. Interventional Radiology", while interventional cardiology, though segregated at most practices, is included for completion.

A note on language:

In general, the studies included in this text were designed by investigators to discern definitive links where possible. These studies have generally stood the test of reproducibility over time, earning them inclusion into this collection. Thus, in many instances this text uses definitive causal terminology (e.g., "reduced", "lowered", etc.) as opposed to associative terminology (e.g., "is linked with a lower risk") to denote strong, time-tested data.

A note on study abbreviations:

While one would benefit greatly from reading this book front-to-back, the summaries stand alone. They are designed so that the reader may look up a study and read one particular summary, and thus we continually redefine abbreviations anew for each individual summary. The choice of abbreviations differ by study and are tailored to individual summaries.

A note on references and indexes:

The e-book edition encourages efficient reading and seamless study. As such, every summarized study has a "clickable" hyperlink near the mid-page which, when "tapped" with the reader's finger, will open the e-reader/tablet/phone internet browser and link directly to the original text by the publishing journal.

This allows the reader to access the original paper instantly (journal subscription and internet access required). The paperback edition includes traditional full text references only. In the e-book edition, a traditional index is replaced by user-searchable text.

CONTRIBUTORS

This text is made possible by the authors and journals that published the original trials as well as the work of numerous contributors at various medical schools and hospitals.

Marc D. Succi, MD | Massachusetts General Hospital

Ravi V. Gottumukkala, MD | Massachusetts General Hospital

Contributing Authors

Benjamin Laguna, MD | University of California San Francisco

Aaron Maxwell, MD | Brown Alpert Medical School

Dylan Wolman, MD | Stanford University

Andrew Cheung, MD | University Health Network, Toronto

Leah H. Carr, MD | Seattle Children's Hospital

Leah Bressler, MD, MPH | Northwestern Memorial Hospital

Dayton McMillan, BSc | Harvard Medical School

David Wang, BSc | University of Toronto School of Medicine

Aliya Ramjaun, BHSc, MSc | University of Toronto School of Medicine

Jimmy Roebker, BSc, MBA | University of Cincinnati School of Medicine

Masis Isikbay, BSc | Harvard Medical School

This page left intentionally blank.

Acknowledgments

This text was compiled with feedback from experts in the field of imaging and intervention. The following expert faculty contributed valuable feedback and/or study suggestions to this text.

Laura L. Avery
Assistant Professor of Radiology, Harvard Medical School
Emergency Imaging Division, Massachusetts General Hospital

Michael A. Blake, MD
Associate Professor of Radiology, Harvard Medical School
Abdominal Imaging Division, Massachusetts General Hospital

David Z. Chow, MD
Instructor in Radiology, Harvard Medical School
Nuclear Medicine Division, Massachusetts General Hospital

Subba R. Digumarthy, MD
Assistant Professor of Radiology, Harvard Medical School
Thoracic Imaging Division, Massachusetts General Hospital

Florian J. Fintelmann, MD
Assistant Professor in Radiology, Harvard Medical School
Thoracic Imaging Division, Massachusetts General Hospital

Efren J. Flores, MD
Instructor in Radiology, Harvard Medical School
Thoracic Imaging Division, Massachusetts General Hospital

Nathan E. Frenk, MD
Clinical Fellow in Radiology, Harvard Medical School
Abdominal Imaging Division, Massachusetts General Hospital

Michael S. Gee, MD PhD
Chief, Pediatric Imaging
Associate Program Director, Diagnostic Radiology Residency
Associate Professor of Radiology, Harvard Medical School
Pediatric Imaging Division, Massachusetts General Hospital

Debra A. Gervais, MD
Division Chief, Abdominal Imaging
Associate Professor of Radiology, Harvard Medical School
Abdominal Imaging Division, Massachusetts General Hospital

Matthew D. Gilman, MD
Associate Director, Thoracic Imaging
Assistant Professor of Radiology, Harvard Medical School
Thoracic Imaging Division, Massachusetts General Hospital

Brian B. Ghoshhajra, MD
Service Chief, Cardiovascular Imaging
Assistant Professor of Radiology, Harvard Medical School
Cardiac Imaging Division, Massachusetts General Hospital

Susanna I. Lee, MD PhD
Chief, Women's' Imaging

Associate Professor of Radiology, Harvard Medical School
Abdominal Imaging Division, Massachusetts General Hospital

Michael H. Lev, MD
Director, Emergency Radiology and Emergency Neuroradiology
Professor of Radiology, Harvard Medical School
Emergency and Neuroradiology Divisions, Massachusetts General Hospital

Umar Mahmood, MD PhD
Professor of Radiology, Harvard Medical School
Nuclear Medicine Division, Massachusetts General Hospital

Theresa C. McLoud, MD
Associate Radiologist in Chief
Program Director, Diagnostic Radiology Residency
Professor of Radiology, Harvard Medical School
Director of Education
Thoracic Imaging Division, Massachusetts General Hospital

Robert A. Novelline, MD
Professor of Radiology, Harvard Medical School
Emergency Imaging Division, Massachusetts General Hospital

Sandra P. Rincon, MD
Assistant Professor of Radiology, Harvard Medical School
Neuroradiology Division, Massachusetts General Hospital

Javier M. Romero, MD
Director, Ultrasound Services
Director, R.H Ackerman Neurovascular Lab
Associate Professor of Radiology, Harvard Medical School
Neuroradiology Division, Massachusetts General Hospital

Dushyant V. Sahani, MD
Associate Professor of Radiology, Harvard Medical School
Abdominal Imaging Division, Massachusetts General Hospital

Jo-Anne O. Shepard. MD
Director, Thoracic Imaging Division
Professor of Radiology, Harvard Medical School
Thoracic Imaging Division, Massachusetts General Hospital

Raul N. Uppot, MD
Assistant Professor of Radiology, Harvard Medical School
Interventional Radiology Division, Massachusetts General Hospital

Jack Wittenberg, MD
Professor of Radiology, Harvard
Medical School
Abdominal Imaging Division,
Massachusetts General Hospital

This page left intentionally blank.

I. Foundational Literature

"The thing that doesn't fit is the thing that's the most interesting, the part that doesn't go according to what you expected."

- Richard P. Feynman, PhD

Fleischner Society Guidelines, 2017 Update: Consolidated follow-up recommendations for incidental solid and subsolid pulmonary nodules

1. The revised Fleischner Society Guidelines (Tables I and II) have reduced the number of unnecessary follow-up examinations required for solid and subsolid nodules and adopted follow-up ranges to provide greater discretion in clinical decision-making.

2. In patients with a low clinical risk for lung cancer, incidentally discovered nodules (solitary or multiple) smaller than 6 mm (<100 mm^3) on computed tomography (CT) do not require additional follow-up; in patients at high risk, an optional CT at 12 months is recommended.

3. No routine follow-up is recommended for ground-glass nodules (GGNs) and part-solid nodules smaller than 6 mm (<100 mm^3); follow-up until 5 years is recommended for those larger than 6 mm (>100 mm^3).

4. Risk factors for malignancy include nodule size, tobacco and other known carcinogens, family history, upper lobe location, emphysema, and pulmonary fibrosis.

Original Date of Publication: March 2017

Study Rundown: The increased use of CT in clinical practice has increased the number of incidentally discovered pulmonary nodules. These nodules can pose diagnostic dilemmas for the radiologist given the wide differential of benign and malignant etiologies. This may result in unnecessary scans and excessive ionizing radiation exposure to patients for nodules with little malignant potential. The original Fleischner Society Guidelines, published in 2005, were evidence-based recommendations regarding follow-up periods for incidentally found solid lung nodules based on size, baseline clinical risk, and nodule morphology. Complementary guidelines for subsolid nodules were issued in 2013 after it was recognized that these unique nodules carried a distinct prognosis. The updated guidelines, published in 2017, incorporate critical new evidence from recent, international, multi-center lung cancer screening trials in its revisions (Table 1). The new evidence is reflected in the following major changes from the original guidelines:

a. For solid nodules, the minimum size threshold that requires routine follow-up has been increased from 4 mm to 6 mm for both high and low-risk patients.
b. Solitary or multiple solid nodules smaller than 6 mm (<100 mm^3) do not require additional follow-up in low risk patients; in high risk patients, an optional CT at 12 months is recommended. Stable solid pulmonary nodules between 6 mm to 8 mm require only one follow-up examination.
c. For solitary part-solid and GGN, a longer initial follow-up period is recommended, and the total duration of follow-up has been increased to 5 years.
d. Follow-up recommendations for both solid and subsolid nodules are provided as a range of time rather than specific time intervals, in order to incorporate various potential clinical risk factors as well as patient preference in determining management.
e. Volumetric thresholds have also been established corresponding to various size criteria for solid and subsolid pulmonary nodules.

Compared to the original guidelines, recent data support a less aggressive approach in the management of small solid and subsolid pulmonary nodules. The Fleischner Society constructed these guidelines based on foundational and recent literature demonstrating several key observations:

1. Patients with solid nodules smaller than 6 mm have been shown to have a cancer risk of less than 1%, even in high-risk patient populations.
2. Volume doubling times for malignant solid pulmonary nodules have been well established in the 100-400-day range, while malignant subsolid nodules may present with a doubling time on the order of 3-5 years.
3. Several clinical and radiologic factors are used for risk stratification and determination of follow-up periods:
    a. Size is a dominant factor in the malignant potential of nodules.
    b. Nodule morphology correlates with malignant likelihood and growth rate (i.e., marginal spiculation and subsolid composition).
    c. Lung cancer occurs more often in the upper lobes, with a preference for the right lung.

d. Emphysema and pulmonary fibrosis (especially idiopathic) are independent risk factors for malignancy.
e. Cigarette smoking portends a greater risk of lethal cancers, increasing in proportion to the degree of smoking.
f. Nodules in cigarette smokers grow faster than in nonsmokers.
g. Malignant risk of nodules increases with patient age.

Low-risk patients are defined as patients with a minimal or absent smoking history and absence of other known risk factors including a history of lung cancer in a first-degree relative, exposure to carcinogenic material (i.e., asbestos, radon, and uranium), upper lobe location, emphysema, or pulmonary fibrosis. Conversely, high-risk patients are defined as patients with a history of smoking or the aforementioned known risk factors.

The guidelines do not apply to patients with known or suspected cancers outside of the lungs, patients younger than 35 years of age, immunocompromised patients, or patients undergoing lung cancer screening. For lung cancer screening, adherence to Lung-RADS (summarized "II. Screening Literature"), a classification system specifically designed for the subset of patients meeting screening eligibility criteria, is recommended.

MacMahon H, Naidich DP, Goo JM, Lee KS, Leung AN, Mayo JR, Mehta AC, Ohno Y, Powell CA, Prokop M, Rubin GD. Guidelines for Management of Incidental Pulmonary Nodules Detected on CT Images: From the Fleischner Society 2017. Radiology. 2017 Feb 23:161659.

Additional Review:

Pinsky PF, Gierada DS, Black W, Munden R, Nath H, Aberle D, et al. Performance of Lung-RADS in the National Lung Screening Trial A Retrospective Assessment Performance of Lung-RADS in the NLST. Ann Intern Med. 2015 Apr 7;162(7):485–91.

Solid Nodules			
	<6 mm (<100 mm^3)	6-8 mm (100-250 mm^3)	>8 mm (>250 mm^3)
Single			
Low Risk	No routine follow-up	CT at 6-12 months, then consider CT at 18-24 months	Consider CT at 3 months, PET/CT, or tissue sampling
High Risk	Optional CT at 12 months	CT at 6-12 months, then CT at 18-24 months	Consider CT at 3 months, PET/CT, or tissue sampling
Multiple			
Low Risk	No routine follow-up	CT at 3-6 months, then consider CT at 18-24 months	CT at 3-6 months, then consider CT at 18-24 months
High Risk	Optional CT at 12 months	CT at 3-6 months, then CT at 18-24 months	CT at 3-6 months, then CT at 18-24 months

Table I. 2017 Fleischner Society Guidelines for Management of Incidentally Detected Solid Pulmonary Nodules in Adults.

Subsolid Nodules		
	<6 mm (<100 mm^3)	≥6 mm (>100 mm^3)
Single		
Ground Glass	No routine follow-up	CT at 6-12 months to confirm persistence, then CT every 2 years until 5 years
Part Solid	No routine follow-up	CT at 3-6 months to confirm persistence. If unchanged and solid component remains <6 mm, annual CT should be performed for 5 years.
Multiple		
Ground Glass or Part Solid	CT at 3-6 months. If stable, consider CT at 2 and 4 years.	CT at 3-6 months. Subsequent management based on the most suspicious nodule(s).

Table II. 2017 Fleischner Society Guidelines for Management of Incidentally Detected Subsolid Pulmonary Nodules in Adults.

Previous Fleischner Society Guidelines, 2013 Update: Frequent CT follow-up recommended for subsolid pulmonary nodules

Previous Fleischner Society Guidelines may still be in use by various practices, so the 2013 and 2005 Guideline summaries are included for reference.

1. In patients with incidentally-detected, solitary, pure ground-glass nodules (GGNs) >5 mm on computed tomography (CT), initial follow-up is recommended at 3 months, followed by annual CT surveillance. Nodules ≤5 mm require no follow-up.

2. In patients with multiple incidentally-detected pure GGNs ≤5 mm, follow-up CT scans at 2 and 4 years is recommended.

3. In patients with incidentally-detected multiple pure GGNs >5 mm without a dominant lesion, follow-up at 3 months with annual CT surveillance is recommended.

4. Solitary part-solid or multiple nodules with a dominant lesion require extended follow-up.

Original Date of Publication: January 2013

Study Rundown: The original Fleischner Society Guidelines for pulmonary nodules, published in 2005, provided guidance for follow-up of solitary pulmonary nodules found incidentally on CT. However, they did not provide specific considerations for a special subset of subsolid or GGNs, nor the presence of multiple nodules. A previous study by Henschke et al. demonstrated that subsolid nodules have an increased risk of malignancy compared to pure solid nodules. The purpose of this landmark guideline from the Fleischner Society was to provide recommendations for imaging follow-up of this unique subset of nodules.

The position statement provided six recommendations for the management of subsolid pulmonary nodules found on CT, detailed in the schematic on the following page. Three are related to solitary subsolid nodules. Specifically, the statement recommends no follow-up for solitary subsolid nodules less than 5 mm in size.

For subsolid nodules greater than 5 mm or for any solitary nodules with both subsolid and solid components, more frequent CT imaging follow-up is required starting at 3 months, followed by yearly CT surveillance for three years. The remaining three recommendations are related to multiple subsolid nodules. For patients with multiple subsolid nodules which are smaller than 5 mm in size, CT follow-up is recommended only at 2 and 4 years. Patients with multiple nodules as well as a dominant lesion (>5 mm) require more frequent follow-up starting at 3 months followed by annual CT surveillance for three years. Finally, in patients with a dominant lesion which contains both subsolid and solid components, increased frequency of follow-up is recommended starting at 3 months, with recommendation for surgical biopsy or resection if the lesion persists and especially if it features a solid component >5 mm.

In addition to the six recommendations, the position statement highlights the importance of using contiguous thin sections (i.e., 1 mm slices) with mediastinal and lung windows to determine the presence of a non-solid component of pulmonary nodules. Additionally, the position statement clarified the use of position emission tomography (PET) in this subgroup as valuable only in the assessment of nodules with both solid and non-solid components greater than 10 mm in size. The recommendations are strengthened by the grading of each specific recommendation based on the quality of the evidence. The updated Fleischner Society Guidelines provide expert opinion based on currently available evidence and have been widely adopted as the imaging follow-up recommendation plan for the management of subsolid pulmonary nodules.

Naidich DP, Bankier AA, MacMahon H, Schaefer-Prokop CM, Pistolesi M, Goo JM, et al. Recommendations for the Management of Subsolid Pulmonary Nodules Detected at CT: A Statement from the Fleischner Society. Radiology. 2013 Jan 1;266(1):304–17.

Additional Review:

Henschke CI, Yankelevitz DF, Mirtcheva R, McGuinness G, McCauley D, Miettinen OS. CT Screening for Lung Cancer. Am J Roentgenol. 2002 May 1;178(5):1053–7.

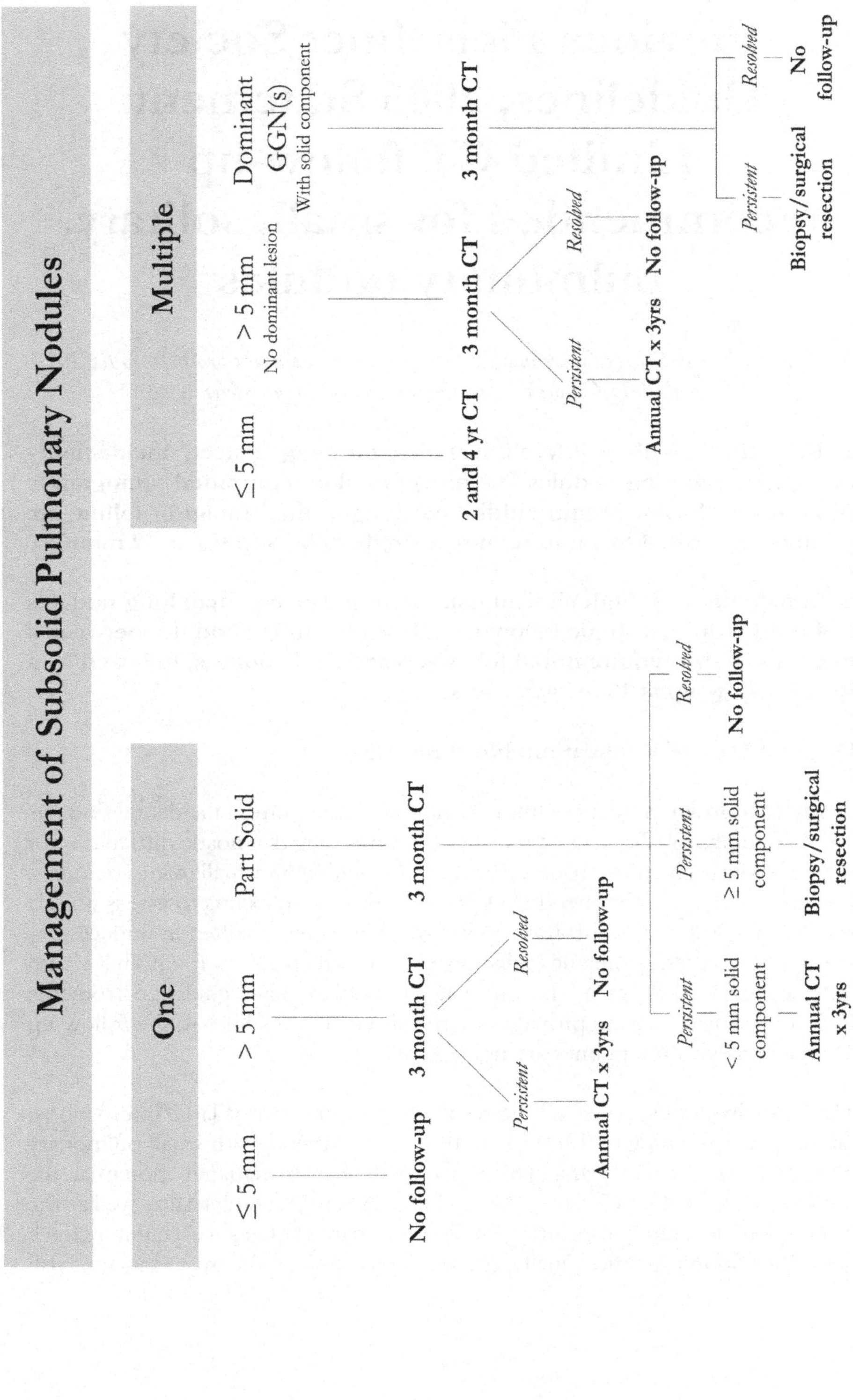

Figure I. 2013 Fleischner Society Guidelines for Subsolid Pulmonary Nodules.

Previous Fleischner Society Guidelines, 2005 Statement: Limited CT follow-up recommended for small, solitary, pulmonary nodules

Previous Fleischner Society Guidelines may still be in use by various practices, so the 2013 and 2005 Guideline summaries are included for reference.

1. In patients with a low clinical risk for lung cancer, incidentally-detected small lung nodules (<4 mm) found on computed tomography (CT) scans do not require additional longitudinal imaging follow-up; nodules between 4 to 6 mm require a single follow-up CT in 12 months.

2. In patients with high clinical risk for lung cancer, small lung nodules (<4 mm) require a single follow-up CT at 12 months; nodules between 4 to 6 mm in size require initial follow-up at 6 to 12 months, followed by a repeat follow-up at 18 to 24 months.

Original Date of Publication: November 2005

Study Rundown: Solitary pulmonary nodules are common incidental findings on radiographs or CT scans of the chest, often posing diagnostic difficulties for the radiologist given the wide differential of benign and malignant etiologies. Earlier guidelines recommended up to 5 CT follow-up exams to assess nodule stability, regardless of morphology or size. This often resulted in unnecessary scans and excessive ionizing radiation exposure to patients for nodules with little malignant potential. The purpose of this landmark guideline from the Fleischner Society was to provide expert-consensus guidelines to the follow-up of incidentally found pulmonary nodules on CT.

The guideline article reviewed the results from a number of large international lung cancer screening trials on the outcomes of patients with small pulmonary nodules. The article highlighted the overall low malignancy potential for nodules between 4 and 7 mm in a large lung cancer screening trial as well as the difficulty in accurately measuring small pulmonary nodules to accurately track growth or doubling time. Finally, the article recognized the importance of risk factors (i.e., smoking status, family history, etc.) in assessing small pulmonary nodules. From this data, the Fleischner Society recommended reducing the overall number of CT follow-ups required for small pulmonary nodules.

The Fleischner Society constructed guidelines based on foundational literature demonstrating several key observations:

a. Half of all smokers 50 years of age or older have at least one nodule at screening.
b. Size is a primary determinant of the malignant potential of nodules.
c. Cigarette smoking portends a greater risk of lethal cancers, increasing in proportion to the degree of smoking.
d. Nodules in cigarette smokers grow faster than in nonsmokers.
e. Nodule morphology correlates with malignant likelihood and growth rate
f. Malignant risk of nodules increases with patient age.

Low-risk patients are defined as patients with a minimal or absent smoking history and absence of other known risk factors including a history of lung cancer in a first degree relative and exposure to carcinogenic material (i.e., asbestos, radon, and uranium). Similarly, high-risk patients are defined as patients with a history of smoking or the aforementioned known risk factors. The guidelines do not apply to patients with known or suspected cancers outside of the lungs, patients younger than 35 years of age, or patients with unexplained fever.

The 2005 Fleischner Society Guidelines are limited in scope to solitary, solid pulmonary nodules and do not provide follow-up recommendations for subsolid nodules or the presence of multiple nodules.

MacMahon H, Austin JHM, Gamsu G, Herold CJ, Jett JR, Naidich DP, et al. Guidelines for Management of Small Pulmonary Nodules Detected on CT Scans: A Statement from the Fleischner Society. Radiology. 2005 Nov 1;237(2):395–400.

Additional Review:

Pinsky PF, Gierada DS, Black W, Munden R, Nath H, Aberle D, et al. Performance of Lung-RADS in the National Lung Screening Trial A Retrospective Assessment Performance of Lung-RADS in the NLST. Ann Intern Med. 2015 Apr 7;162(7):485–91.

Nodule size	Low-Risk Patient	High-Risk Patient
≤4 mm	– No follow up	– 12 month CT – If stable, no further follow-up
>4 mm - 6 mm	– 12 month CT – If stable, no further follow-up	– 6-12 month CT – If stable, repeat CT at 18-24 months
>6 mm - 8 mm	– 6-12 month CT – If stable, repeat CT at 18-24 months	– 3-6 month CT – If stable, repeat CT at 9-12 months and 24 months
>8 mm	– CT at 3, 9, and 24 months – Consider dynamic contrast-enhanced CT, PET or biopsy	– CT at 3, 9, and 24 months – Consider dynamic contrast-enhanced CT, PET or biopsy

Table I. 2005 Fleischner Society Guidelines for Solid Pulmonary Nodules.

CT insensitive to mediastinal lymph node metastasis in bronchogenic carcinoma

1. Computed tomography (CT) of the chest is limited in the ability to detect the presence of mediastinal lymph node involvement in patients with bronchogenic carcinoma.

2. This study helped popularize the use of 1 cm (measured in short axis) as the criteria for abnormally enlarged lymph nodes.

Original Date of Publication: February 1992

Study Rundown: Lung cancer is the leading cause of cancer-related death worldwide with over 1.2 million deaths in 2012. Accurate evaluation of mediastinal lymphadenopathy is vital in the staging of a patient with lung cancer to provide prognostic information for patients as well as to direct treatment. CT scans of the chest provide visualization of mediastinal lymph nodes not typically accessible by mediastinoscopy or thoracotomy; however, there have been conflicting reports on the sensitivity and specificity of chest CT to identify lymph node metastases in the mediastinum. The purpose of this landmark prospective trial was to determine the accuracy of chest CT to identify mediastinal lymph node metastases in patients with lung cancer.

The trial prospectively followed over 140 patients with bronchogenic carcinoma that underwent chest CT evaluation with surgical staging correlation. CT evidence of mediastinal metastases was defined as any lymph nodes greater than 1 cm in short axis. At the conclusion of the trial, the sensitivity and specificity of CT examinations for mediastinal metastases were found to be 64% and 62%, respectively. Additionally, the sensitivity for individual nodal stations within the mediastinum was lower at 44%. In particular, there were high rates of false-positive lymph nodes within the right paratracheal group and the aorticopulmonary window. Although larger nodes were associated with increased likelihood of mediastinal metastases, over one-third of all lymph nodes over 2 cm were found to be benign and hyperplastic. The results of this study demonstrated the relative insensitivity of CT to identify mediastinal metastases in patients with lung cancer due to confounding conditions such as atelectasis or pneumonitis leading to hyperplastic and reactive lymph node changes. This landmark trial provides strong evidence for the use of chest CT scans in conjunction with mediastinoscopy or thoracotomy to adequately provide staging information for patients with bronchogenic carcinoma.

In-Depth [prospective cohort]: This was a prospective study of 143 patients with pathologically-confirmed, non-small cell lung cancer from a single institution in the United States. Each patient underwent CT examination of the chest followed by pathological staging of the mediastinum either through mediastinoscopy or thoracotomy. Mediastinal lymph nodes were measured in the short axis and considered abnormal if they measured greater than 1 cm in diameter. The primary outcome of interest was the patient-by-patient accuracy rate of the CT findings correlated with the pathological results from surgical staging. Secondary outcomes included the accuracy of each specific mediastinal nodal station, as defined by the American Thoracic Society mapping scheme, to its pathological correlate. Overall, 401 mediastinal lymph nodes were evaluated, of which 369 (83%) were found to be normal. At the conclusion of the trial, the CT sensitivity for mediastinal metastases for each individual patient was 64% with a specificity of 62%. The sensitivity and specificity for all nodal stations are 44% and 85%, respectively. In the subgroup analysis of each individual lymph node station, groups 4R, 5, and 10R in the right paratracheal and aorticopulmonary window demonstrated the highest false-positive rate. Increase in lymph node size on CT was associated with an increased likelihood of metastatic disease; however, over 33% of the lymph nodes between 2 and 4 cm in size in this cohort demonstrated a benign hyperplastic reaction rather than metastasis. For lymph nodes <1 cm in short axis diameter, the prevalence of metastases was 13%; for nodes 1 – 1.9 cm, the prevalence of metastases was 25%; for nodes 2.0 – 2.9 cm, the prevalence of metastases was 62%.

McLoud TC, Bourgouin PM, Greenberg RW, Kosiuk JP, Templeton PA, Shepard JA, et al. Bronchogenic carcinoma: analysis of staging in the mediastinum with CT by correlative lymph node mapping and sampling. Radiology. 1992 Feb 1;182(2):319–23.

CT-guided percutaneous lung biopsies more effective for larger pulmonary nodules

1. Computed tomography (CT)-guided percutaneous lung biopsies demonstrated a significantly higher accuracy for pulmonary nodules greater than 1.5 cm in diameter compared to small pulmonary nodules (<1.5 cm).

2. There were no significant differences in the rates of complications for either large or small pulmonary nodules.

Original Date of Publication: July 1996

Study Rundown: CT-guided percutaneous needle aspiration lung biopsy provides a minimally-invasive method of distinguishing benign and malignant lung lesions. However, this procedure may be associated with an increased risk of complications, including pneumothorax, air embolism, and inadequate sampling leading to false-negative results. The purpose of this landmark retrospective review was to explore the differences in diagnostic accuracy as well as the complication rates for CT-guided percutaneous needle aspiration biopsies between small (<1.5 cm) versus large (>1.5 cm) lung nodules.

This trial retrospectively reviewed the outcomes of 97 consecutive patients that underwent CT-guided percutaneous needle aspiration of a lung mass. At the conclusion of the trial, the diagnostic accuracy of needle aspiration was high for both small and large pulmonary nodules; however, percutaneous biopsies of larger nodules demonstrated significantly higher diagnostic accuracy and overall sensitivity compared to small nodules. Furthermore, small pulmonary nodules had a higher false-negative rate compared to large nodules. With respect to procedural complications, there were no significant differences in the rates of pneumothorax between patients with small and large lung nodules, with an overall low number requiring chest tube placement.

This trial demonstrated that CT-guided percutaneous needle aspiration was safe and had an acceptable accuracy for both large and small pulmonary nodules; however, biopsy of small nodules resulted in a significantly lower accuracy. Additionally, the high false-negative rate for small nodules indicates that a negative result may be of limited clinical value. The results of this trial support the use of additional biopsy procedures for negative percutaneous results. Furthermore, although the size cut-off in this trial was 1.5 cm, most large pulmonary nodules in the study were larger than 3 cm. The majority of subsequent studies on percutaneous lung biopsies have used 3 cm as the cut-off for small pulmonary nodules.

In-Depth [retrospective cohort]: This study included 97 consecutive patients that underwent CT-guided percutaneous needle aspiration lung biopsy in a single center. The primary outcome was the diagnostic accuracy and safety of CT-guided lung biopsies. All biopsies were performed by chest radiologists, chest radiology fellows, or radiology residents under the supervision of attending radiologists. Overall, 27 small nodules (mean size: 1.15 cm; range: 0.4 to 1.5 cm) and 70 large nodules (mean size: 3.17 cm; range: 1.6 to 8.2 cm) were biopsied. All biopsy specimens were correlated with pathologic findings from surgery. At the conclusion of the trial, 23 of 27 (85%) small nodules and 62 of 70 (89%) large nodules were found to be malignant. Biopsy of large pulmonary nodules demonstrated a significantly higher sensitivity (94% versus 72%; $p < 0.05$) and accuracy (96% versus 74%; $p < 0.05$) compared to small nodules. There were no differences in specificity between large and small nodule biopsy. There were similar rates of pneumothorax for patients with both small and large pulmonary nodules. There were no post-procedural fatalities in either group.

Li H, Boiselle PM, Shepard JO, Trotman-Dickenson B, McLoud TC. Diagnostic accuracy and safety of CT-guided percutaneous needle aspiration biopsy of the lung: comparison of small and large pulmonary nodules. Am J Roentgenol. 1996 Jul 1;167(1):105–9.

The PIOPED II trial: CT sensitive and specific for pulmonary embolism

1. Multidetector computed tomographic angiography (CTA) was highly sensitive and specific for the diagnosis of pulmonary embolism (PE) when compared to a composite reference standard.

2. When combined with computed tomographic venography (CTV), sensitivity was increased without a significant increase in the specificity, positive predictive value, or negative predictive value.

Original Date of Publication: June 2006

Study Rundown: PE refers to the blockage of one or more arteries within the lung by a blood clot or other substance that originated within another part of the body. It is a commonly considered diagnosis among patients presenting to the emergency department with shortness of breath and chest pain, and failure to diagnose PE is associated with significant mortality. Historically, the diagnosis was made by the introduction of contrast material directly into the pulmonary arteries by a catheter. This technique was replaced by ventilation-perfusion (VQ) scanning, which compares patterns of blood flow and oxygenation in the lung using a radioactive tracer. Though significantly less invasive, VQ scanning was often difficult to interpret and was itself replaced by CTA beginning in the 1980s and 1990s.

Early reports of the diagnostic performance of CTA were generally positive but mixed, and the optimal method for evaluating patients with suspected PE initially remained uncertain. In the second Prospective Investigation of Pulmonary Embolism Diagnosis (PIOPED II) trial, CTA with and without concomitant lower extremity CTV was compared with a composite reference standard including both VQ scanning and conventional angiography. The results of this trial showed that both CTA and combined CTA-CTV were highly sensitive and specific for the diagnosis of PE, and that the combination of clinical judgment with the results from CTA or CTA-CTV evaluation was sufficient to accurately rule-in and rule-out PE in the vast majority of patients.

In-Depth [prospective cohort]: This prospective trial was conducted at 8 clinic sites throughout North America. All adult patients with signs and symptoms concerning for acute PE who were referred for evaluation were consecutively screened for enrollment (n=7284). Both inpatients and outpatients were considered. Key exclusion criteria included anticoagulant use, hemodialysis, critical illness, patients on ventilators, and recent myocardial infarction. Following screening and consent, all enrolled patients (n=1090) underwent combined CTA-CTV, as well as one or more of the components that together formed the composite reference standard. This included VQ scanning, lower extremity venous ultrasonography with Doppler imaging, and, when necessary, digital subtraction angiography (DSA) of the pulmonary arteries. All imaging studies were reviewed by 2 blinded radiologists unaffiliated with the clinical sites, with additional radiologists serving as arbiters in the event of discordant interpretations. Patients were considered to have a positive CTA if there was any partial or complete filling defect identified within one or more pulmonary arteries, and a positive CTV if there was any partial or complete filling defect identified within one of the lower extremity veins. Using the composite reference standard, patients were diagnosed with PE if any of the following conditions were met: high probability VQ scan in a patient without a history of PE; filling defect on pulmonary DSA; or visualized lower extremity clot by ultrasound.

A total of 824 patients (mean age 51.7±17.1 years; 62% women; 89% outpatient) successfully completed both CTA-CTV and the composite reference standard. Among this cohort, 192 PEs were diagnosed. For those with diagnostic-quality CTA alone (773 patients, 94%), the sensitivity was 83% and the specificity was 96%, while the positive and negative predictive values were 86% and 95%, respectively. Considering those patients with diagnostic-quality combined CTA-CTV (737 patients, 89%) separately, the sensitivity was 90% and the specificity was 95%, while the positive and negative predictive values were 85% and 97%, respectively. The results varied substantially by clinical suspicion, with a positive predictive value of 96% among those with a high pre-test probability of PE and a positive predictive value of 58% among those with a low-pretest probability. Complications associated with CTA-CTV were rare and included mild allergic reactions and transiently increased creatinine.

Stein PD, Fowler SE, Goodman LR, Gottschalk A, Hales CA, Hull RD, et al. Multidetector Computed Tomography for Acute Pulmonary Embolism. The New England Journal of Medicine. 2006 Jun 1;354(22):2317–27.

The ROMICAT 1 trial: Coronary computed tomographic angiography highly sensitive for acute coronary syndrome in patients with acute chest pain

1. In patients presenting with chest pain and a low to intermediate risk of acute coronary syndrome (ACS), computed tomographic coronary angiography (CTCA) demonstrated high sensitivity and negative predictive value for acute coronary syndrome.

Original Date of Publication: May 2009

Study Rundown: Chest pain is one of the most common patient complaints and accounts for over 100 million emergency department visits every year in the U.S. alone. Most patients presenting with chest pain have not suffered an ACS, though many are admitted to hospital for further monitoring and testing. CTCA is a rapid test that can identify significant stenoses in the coronary arteries, though its utility in chest pain evaluation was unclear at the time of this study, having only been assessed in several small studies.

The Rule Out Myocardial Infarction using Computer Assisted Tomography 1 (ROMICAT 1) trial was a blinded prospective cohort study that sought to determine whether CTCA was useful in assessing patients with acute chest pain and low to intermediate risk of ACS. The absence of coronary artery disease on CTCA demonstrated a sensitivity of 100% and a negative predictive value (NPV) of 100% for ACS. Thus, CTCA may be of high utility in evaluating patients with chest pain in the emergency department and facilitate more rapid discharge of patients with low to intermediate likelihood of ACS. Additional radiation exposure remains one of the limitations inherent in this technology, though decreasingly so with modern techniques including prospective electrocardiogram (ECG) triggering.

In-Depth [prospective cohort]: This study examined 368 patients who were >18 years of age, presented to the emergency department with chest pain lasting >5 minutes in the previous 24 hours, had initially normal troponin levels and ECG, were suspected to have ischemic chest pain, were admitted to the hospital to rule out myocardial infarction (MI), and were able to perform a breath hold of 10-15 seconds. Exclusion criteria included initial elevation in troponin or CK-MB levels, new diagnostic ECG changes (ST-segment elevation or depression ≥1 mm or T wave inversions >4 mm in 2 contiguous leads), hemodynamic or clinical instability, known allergy to iodinated contrast, and history of established coronary artery disease (previous stent implantation or coronary bypass grafting).

CT imaging was performed using a 64-slice scanner (Sensation 64, Siemens Medical Solutions) with iodinated contrast. Patients with a heart rate >60 beats/min received intravenous metoprolol 5-20 mg, unless their systolic blood pressure was <100 mmHg. Axial images were reconstructed using a retrospectively ECG-gated algorithm. The presence of significant coronary artery stenosis was defined as any luminal obstruction >50% in any coronary segment.

By CTCA, 183 patients (50%) were found to have no coronary disease. In this cohort, identifying no plaque demonstrated a sensitivity and NPV of 100% (95%CI 89-100%) and 100% (95%CI 98-100%), respectively, for ACS. Finding any plaque yielded a specificity of 54% (95%CI 49-60%) for ACS with a positive predictive value (PPV) of 17%. The absence of significant coronary stenosis demonstrated a sensitivity of 77% (95%CI 59-90%) and a NPV of 98%, while the presence of coronary stenosis demonstrated a specificity of 87% (95%CI 83-90%) and a PPV of 35%. Additionally, both plaque and stenosis, as assessed on CTA, predicted ACS independent of cardiovascular risk factors or TIMI risk score (AUC 0.88, 0.82 versus 0.63, respectively; all $p < 0.05$).

Hoffmann U, Bamberg F, Chae CU, Nichols JH, Rogers IS, Seneviratne SK, et al. Coronary Computed Tomography Angiography for Early Triage of Patients With Acute Chest PainThe ROMICAT (Rule Out Myocardial Infarction using Computer Assisted Tomography) Trial. J Am Coll Cardiol. 2009 May 5;53(18):1642–50.

The ROMICAT 2 trial: Coronary computed tomographic angiography shortens hospital stays for acute chest pain

1. In patients presenting to the emergency department with acute chest pain, evaluation with computed tomographic coronary angiography (CTCA) led to significantly shorter hospital stays compared to the standard care without CTCA.

2. There were no undetected acute coronary syndromes (ACSs) in either group, and no significant difference between the groups in the rate of major adverse cardiovascular events (MACE) at 28 days.

Original Date of Publication: July 2012

Study Rundown: The Rule Out Myocardial Infarction/Ischemia Using Computer Assisted Tomography 1 (ROMICAT 1) trial was a prospective cohort study that demonstrated the high sensitivity and negative predictive value of CTCA in patients with low to intermediate risk of ACS. The ROMICAT 2 trial was a randomized controlled trial that compared a strategy incorporating CTCA with standard care in assessing patients presenting to the emergency department with chest pain. Patients in the CTCA group experienced significantly shorter hospital stays and higher rates of direct discharge from the emergency department compared to those receiving standard care. Moreover, there were no cases of undetected ACS in either group, and no significant difference in the rate of major adverse cardiovascular events (MACE) at 28 days after the index visit.

In-Depth [randomized controlled trial]: The study involved 1000 patients recruited from 9 centers across the U.S. who were randomized in a 1:1 ratio to evaluation involving CTCA or to standard evaluation. Patients were eligible for the trial if they were 40-74 years of age, had chest pain or an angina equivalent lasting >5 minutes in the 24 hours prior to presenting, and warranted further risk stratification to rule out acute coronary syndrome (ACS) according to the assessing physician. Exclusion criteria included history of known coronary artery disease, new diagnostic ischemic changes on the initial electrocardiogram

(ECG), initial elevated troponin, creatinine >132.6 µmol/L (>1.5 mg/dL), iodine contrast allergy, and body mass index >40.

At least 64-slice CT technology was required, and both retrospectively ECG-gated and prospectively ECG-triggered CTCAs were allowed. The primary endpoint was length of hospital stay. Secondary endpoints included time to diagnosis, rate of direct discharge from the emergency department, and resource utilization. The secondary safety endpoints were undetected ACS and MACE (death, myocardial infarction, unstable angina, or urgent coronary revascularization) within 28 days, and periprocedural complications (stroke, bleeding, anaphylaxis, renal failure).

The mean length of hospitalization was 7.6 hours shorter for patients in the CTA group compared to those undergoing standard evaluation ($p < 0.001$). Patients undergoing CTCA also experienced significantly shorter time to diagnosis ($p < 0.001$), and had significantly higher rates of direct discharge from the emergency department (47% versus 12%, $p < 0.001$). There were no undetected ACSs and no significant differences between the groups in the rate of MACE at 28 days ($p = 0.18$) or periprocedural complications ($p = 0.50$).

Patients in the CTA group had significantly higher rates of diagnostic testing ($p < 0.001$) and functional testing ($p < 0.001$) than those in the standard group. Moreover, there was a trend towards higher rates of coronary angiography ($p = 0.06$) and revascularization ($p = 0.16$) in those who underwent CTCA, though the costs of care were not significantly different between the two groups for the index visit and follow-up period ($p = 0.65$).

Hoffmann U, Truong QA, Schoenfeld DA, Chou ET, Woodard PK, Nagurney JT, et al. Coronary CT Angiography versus Standard Evaluation in Acute Chest Pain. The New England Journal of Medicine. 2012 Jul 26;367(4):299–308.

Breast ultrasound sensitive for cancer and carries a low false positive rate

1. In a large cohort of women referred for evaluation of one or more solid breast lesions, ultrasound (US) showed a sensitivity of 98.4% for malignancy and was associated with a negative predictive value of 99.5%.

Original Date of Publication: July 1995

Study Rundown: At the time of this study, US was used to help identify simple breast cysts, a common and benign finding that can initially generate concern when identified on mammography. Given the success of US in this area, numerous attempts were made to expand the technology's use to include other indeterminate breast lesions, particularly solid masses. Initial studies were unsupportive, however, and multiple guideline sets were published explicitly recommending against the use of US for solid breast mass evaluation.

Given dramatic improvements in the resolution and functional capabilities of US, however, this issue was revisited in 1995 with publication of this prospective trial. A large cohort of women with suspicious breast lesions referred for breast US were evaluated over several years. Only women with solid lesions were considered. All women underwent biopsy following their US, and biopsy and imaging results were compared to determine the diagnostic performance of US. Results revealed that, contrary to prior data, US was highly sensitive for malignancy in solid breast masses. Conversely, in the absence of concerning imaging features, US appropriately excluded malignancy with few diagnostic errors. Strengths of the trial included its prospective methodology, the large number of patients successfully enrolled, and the low attrition rate. The primary limitations of the trial included heterogeneous biopsy methods and the inherent variability associated with subjective rating scales. Today, breast US remains a substantial component of the breast imager's toolkit and is routinely used for solid breast mass evaluation.

In-Depth [prospective cohort]: A total of 662 patients (mean age 47 years) with suspicious breast lesions were prospectively enrolled over an approximately 4-year period following referral for breast US. The most common reason for referral was an antecedent abnormal mammogram. A total of 750 solid nodules were evaluated by US. Studies were blindly interpreted by 5 breast radiologists and findings were classified as "benign" or "malignant" based on the presence or absence of several previously-published imaging features. When no features were present, a classification of "indeterminate" was made. When available, initial mammograms and their interpretations were also reviewed. All enrolled patients subsequently underwent either core needle or excisional biopsy for definitive pathologic diagnosis. These final diagnoses were compared with imaging results to determine the diagnostic performance of US in the evaluation of suspicious solid breast lesions.

Pathologic examination revealed 625 (83%) benign nodules and 125 (17%) malignant nodules. The most common malignant lesion was infiltrating ductal adenocarcinoma, and the most common benign lesion was fibroadenoma. One hundred (73%) of the 137 malignant nodules were correctly diagnosed by US. The overall sensitivity and specificity for breast US in the detection of malignancy were 98.4% and 67.8%, respectively. Due to a high false positive rate, the positive predictive value was 38%, while the negative predictive value was 99.5%, with only 2 false positive examinations. Twenty-seven nodules that were interpreted as malignant or indeterminate by US had been previously interpreted as definitively or probably benign by mammography. An additional 44 nodules accurately interpreted as malignant by US were interpreted as indeterminate by mammography. The US features most strongly associated with malignancy were spiculation (OR 5.5), taller-than-wider shape (OR 4.9), and angular margins (OR 4.0).

Stavros AT, Thickman D, Rapp CL, Dennis MA, Parker SH, Sisney GA. Solid breast nodules: use of sonography to distinguish between benign and malignant lesions. Radiology. *1995 Jul 1;196(1):123–34.*

Breast density increases the risk of cancer and hinders mammographic detection

1. Women with mammographic density obscuring more than 75% of the imaged breast demonstrated a significantly increased risk of breast cancer detected either by screening or within 12 months of a negative screening examination, compared to those with density in less than 10% of the mammogram.

2. The increase in risk of breast cancer in women with dense breasts was greatest in younger women. In this demographic, 25% of all detected cancers were attributable to density in at least 50% of the mammogram.

Original Date of Publication: January 2007

Study Rundown: As the relative proportion between fat and epithelial and stromal tissues shifts away from fat, the breast becomes increasingly "dense" on mammography. As many tumors may also appear radiodense, they may be hidden by the predominance of stroma within a dense breast, subsequently hindering early detection, while that increased density may itself be a risk factor for oncogenesis. Unfortunately, this interaction between breast density and the ability to detect cancers on screening previously confounded research regarding the risks associated with mammographic density. Cancer risk would be underestimated if based solely on those tumors detected at screening due to an omission of those masked by breast density, while risk would be overestimated if based solely on cancers detected by alternate means, as it would focus only on those missed at screening.

The present study attempted to better estimate the true risk of mammographic density as it relates to breast cancer by determining the risk both at the time of screening and thereafter among women with quantified breast density from three large national case-control studies. Women with density in 75% or more of the mammogram demonstrated a significantly increased risk of breast cancer compared to those with density in 10% or less of the mammogram both at the time of screening or by alternate means. This risk was found to persist for up to 8 years after initial screening. The attributable risk of cancer to breast density was most marked in younger women, for whom 26% of all detected cancers, and 50% of those detected within 1 year of a negative examination were attributable to density in at least 50% of the mammogram. This study established an accurate estimate of the incidence of breast cancers attributable to increased breast density by combining those data for those detected at screening and those detected up to 12 months after a negative screening examination, representing cancers likely present at the time of initial screening but obscured by mammographic density.

In-Depth [case-control study]: This retrospective case-control study pooled data from three large mammographic screening programs in Canada, the National Breast Screening Study (NBSS), the Ontario Breast Screening Program (OBSP), and the Screening Mammography Program of British Columbia (SMPBC.) A total of 1114 case-control pairs were included (mean age 56.7±9.1 years). Case subjects had histologically verified invasive breast cancer, excluding those with cancers detected within 12 months of their first screening mammogram, while up to 10 control subjects were matched to each index case on the basis of age, body-mass index, pregnancy and menopause history, hormone-replacement use, family history of breast cancer, and quantification of mammographic density. Mammograms from each subject were submitted and independently classified into one of six quantified degrees of breast density (0%, <10%, 10 to <25%, 25 to <50%, 50 to <75%, and ≥75%) by two radiologists and a single observer using a computer-assisted technique.

Notably, the average percentage of mammographic density was 5.8% higher among case subjects than control subjects at baseline. Women below the median age of 56 years were 3 times more likely to have breasts with a mammographic density of ≥50%. The combined odds ratio for the detection of breast cancer among women with ≥75% mammographic density was 4.7 (95%CI 3.0-7.4) as compared to those with ≤10% density. For those cancers detected at screening, the odds ratio was 3.5 (95%CI 2.0-6.2), while it was 17.8 (95%CI 4.8-65.9) for those cancers detected within 12 months of a negative screening mammogram. For cancers detected over a year after the last negative screening mammogram, the odds ratio was 5.7 (95%CI 2.1-15.5). These increased risks were significantly associated with percentage of breast density at all time periods, up to 8 years after entry into the study ($p < 0.001$). The attributable risk of breast cancer for a mammographic density of ≥50% was 16% for all cancers, much of which was limited to the 12 months following screening, suggesting that tumor masking was the principal mechanism of risk, rather than rapid tumor growth.

Boyd NF, Guo H, Marin LJ, Sun L, Stone J, Fishell E, et al. Mammographic Density and the Risk and Detection of Breast Cancer. The New England Journal of Medicine. 2007 Jan 18;356(3):227–36.

MRI enhances diagnostic certainty of ovarian cancer following indeterminate ultrasound

1. In women with an indeterminate ovarian mass on ultrasonography, magnetic resonance imaging (MRI) provided a significantly higher change in post-test probability compared to computed tomography (CT) or Doppler ultrasound.

Original Date of Publication: July 2005

Study Rundown: Ovarian cancer is the second most common gynecological malignancy with a world-wide incidence of 11.9 cases per 100 000 women. Accurate diagnosis of patients presenting with adnexal masses is crucial to allow timely surgical diagnosis and intervention. Although ultrasound is the first-line imaging modality in women for assessment of a suspicious adnexal mass, at the time of this study there was no evidence-based consensus on the management options for patients following an indeterminate adnexal mass on ultrasonography. The purpose of this landmark meta-analysis was to determine the optimal second-line imaging modality to assess an indeterminate ovarian mass on ultrasound for both pre- and post-menopausal women.

The authors performed a literature review to determine the prevalence of ovarian cancer in patients presenting with an adnexal mass as well as the sensitivity and specificity of Doppler ultrasound, CT, and MRI in the characterization of adnexal masses following ultrasonography. The change in pre- and post-test probabilities was calculated for each imaging modality. At the conclusion of the study, the use of any additional imaging modalities was associated with a significant increase in post-test probability for both pre- and post-menopausal women. However, MRI demonstrated significantly higher diagnostic certainty in post-test probability for ovarian cancer compared to Doppler US or CT in both pre- and post-menopausal women. The positive likelihood ratio for contrast-enhanced MRI was 10-fold higher than Doppler US and approximately 7-fold higher than CT. The results of this trial demonstrate that in both pre- and post-menopausal women with an indeterminate ovarian mass on ultrasonography, second-line imaging is warranted to improve diagnostic certainty for ovarian cancer. Additionally, MRI is the ideal second line imaging modality and provides a significantly higher level of diagnostic certainty in comparison to Doppler US or CT.

The study was limited by the absence of integration of serum CA-125 into the diagnostic algorithm of adnexal masses, which may have improved diagnostic certainty. Nevertheless, this study served to inform the use of MRI as the second line imaging modality to determine the need for surgical evaluation of suspected ovarian cancer in both pre- and post-menopausal women.

In-Depth [meta-analysis]: The authors performed a literature review of English-language studies using the MEDLINE database to determine the pre-test probability of ovarian cancer in pre- and post-menopausal women. The authors performed a literature review of 83 articles which met the following inclusion criteria: 1) presence of adnexal mass not detected during screening; 2) availability of histopathological information. Two experienced readers abstracted data from each article and disagreements were resolved with consensus. A similar methodology was utilized for a literature review of 12 articles to determine the sensitivity and specificity of ovarian mass characterization by Doppler US, CT, and MRI. Positive and negative likelihood ratios were calculated from the average weighted means of sensitivity and specificity. At the conclusion of the study, the post-test probability following an indeterminate US result was 25% and 63% for pre- and post-menopausal women, respectively. Robust negative LR following initial indeterminate US result were seen for Doppler US (0.19), CT (0.22), and contrast-enhanced MRI (0.2). With respect to positive LR, contrast-enhanced MRI (44.2) was significantly more robust compared to Doppler US (4.69) and CT (6.81). This effect was seen in both pre- and post-menopausal women.

Kinkel K, Lu Y, Mehdizade A, Pelte M-F, Hricak H. Indeterminate Ovarian Mass at US: Incremental Value of Second Imaging Test for Characterization—Meta-Analysis and Bayesian Analysis. Radiology. 2005 Jul 1;236(1):85–94.

Non-contrast CT sensitive and specific for kidney stones

1. Among patients with acute flank pain, non-contrast computed tomography (CT) of the abdomen and pelvis demonstrated a sensitivity of 97% and a specificity of 96% for the diagnosis of kidney stones.

2. Non-contrast CT was associated with a low false negative rate and suggested alternative diagnoses in a significant number of patients without evidence of kidney stones, thus increasing the overall diagnostic yield.

Original Date of Publication: January 1996

Study Rundown: Kidney stones, or nephrolithiasis, are a common cause of pain among patients presenting to the emergency department. Historically, the evaluation of patients with suspected nephrolithiasis consisted of plain radiographs together with clinical history, physical examination, and laboratory data. However, this combination was associated with a high false negative rate. The diagnostic yield was improved with the widespread adoption of intravenous pyelography (IP), a fluoroscopic technique in which dye is introduced into the urinary tract and imaged by x-rays in real-time. The use of IP improved stone detection but was associated with higher radiation exposure and the need for contrast administration, and the false negative rate remained high. There remained a significant need for a fast, accurate diagnostic technique among patients with suspected stone disease. With the introduction of CT into standard practice, there was a strong push towards its adoption as the standard for evaluation of nephrolithiasis given its high spatial and contrast resolution.

In the present study, patients with symptoms concerning for nephrolithiasis were imaged with non-contrast CT of the abdomen and pelvis to determine the presence or absence of stones within the urinary tract. These patients then underwent a combination of repeat imaging, surgery, or close clinical follow-up to determine the final diagnosis. The results suggested that non-contrast CT was highly sensitive and specific for nephrolithiasis and was associated with few false negative findings. Moreover, because of the ability to image other structures within the abdomen and pelvis in high resolution, CT was able to identify possible alternative diagnoses, such as appendicitis or infection, in nearly 33% of patients without evidence of stones. The study was limited by the use of a composite reference standard and the lack of outcome data. Today, non-contrast CT in conjunction with ultrasonography remains the diagnostic gold standard among patients with suspected kidney stones.

In-Depth [prospective cohort]: A total of 292 consecutive patients referred for evaluation of possible nephrolithiasis at a single center underwent non-contrast CT of the abdomen and pelvis by standard protocol. Images were blindly reviewed by 2 radiologists with expertise in CT interpretation, and imaging diagnoses were made by consensus. Findings considered positive for nephrolithiasis included direct visualization of a stone within the ureters or bladder or unilateral collecting system dilation and perinephric stranding without direct stone visualization. Of the original cohort that underwent imaging, 210 patients (98 male, 112 female; age range 18-85 years) went on to have diagnostic confirmation in the form of surgery, repeat imaging, or clinical follow-up. The results of the study suggested a sensitivity and negative predictive value of 97%, and a specificity and positive predictive value of 96%. The overall diagnostic accuracy of non-contrast CT in the evaluation of patients with suspected nephrolithiasis was 97%. Thirty-one patients without evidence of stone disease on CT (27.6%) were found to have an unsuspected extra-renal abnormality, the most common of which was a symptomatic adnexal mass.

Smith RC, Verga M, McCarthy S, Rosenfield AT. Diagnosis of acute flank pain: value of unenhanced helical CT. American Journal of Roentgenology. 1996 Jan 1;166(1):97–101.

CT not sufficient to rule out early subarachnoid hemorrhage

1. In a retrospective review of 119 patients with subarachnoid hemorrhage (SAH), computed tomography (CT) scan within 12 hours of symptom onset failed to identify the presence of hemorrhage in two patients.

2. Lumbar puncture 12 hours after symptom onset definitively diagnosed all patients with SAH.

Original Date of Publication: March 1995

Study Rundown: SAH is most commonly due to a ruptured saccular aneurysm and is associated with high rates of mortality and significant neurologic morbidity. Although non-contrast CT scans provide high sensitivity in detection of SAH within 24 hours, given the significant morbidity associated with a missed diagnosis, definitive diagnosis by lumbar puncture is generally recommended when a CT scan is negative. The purpose of this landmark retrospective study was to assess whether a non-contrast CT within 12 hours after symptom onset can identify SAH and remove the need for lumbar puncture.

Of 175 retrospectively reviewed patients presenting with acute headache, 119 consecutive patients with lumbar puncture-confirmed SAH received a CT scan within 12 hours of presentation. At the conclusion of the study, there was evidence of subarachnoid blood on CT in 117 cases. Two cases of SAH were reported normal on CT with no evidence of blood or other abnormalities on repeat interpretation. Both cases underwent angiography which demonstrated a culprit aneurysm in the posterior inferior cerebellar artery (PICA) and posterior communicating artery (PCA), respectively. The results of this study demonstrated that CT scan cannot definitively rule out SAH in patients who present within 12 hours after onset of symptoms. Therefore, further diagnostic testing with lumbar puncture to evaluate for xanthochromia is recommended in patients with normal head CT scans. This study was one of the first studies to demonstrate the diagnostic accuracy of CT for SAH detection in patients who present early after symptom onset. Although a recent study by Cortnum et al. suggested that improved detection with modern CT scanners may obviate the need for lumbar puncture in this setting, the results of the study by Van Der Wee et al. have still been used to inform recent guidelines from the

American Stroke Association which continue to recommend the use of lumbar puncture in patients suspected of having SAH with a normal CT head examination.

In-Depth [retrospective cohort]: This study retrospectively reviewed outcomes of 175 patients who presented to two hospitals in the Netherlands with acute headache between 1989 and 1993. Patients were excluded if they had any focal neurological deficits or if their CT scan was performed greater than 12 hours after the onset of symptoms. The CT scans were assessed by a neuroradiologist and two neurologists. The primary outcome was the accuracy of CT scans in detecting the presence of SAH. At the conclusion of the study, 117 (67%) patients demonstrated evidence of SAH on CT. However, lumbar puncture identified two patients (2%) with SAH that had normal CT scans. These two patients were found to have a PICA aneurysm and PCA aneurysm, respectively. Of the 117 patients with CT evidence of SAH, the distribution of etiologies consisted of ruptured aneurysm arising from the anterior cerebral artery (n=29), internal carotid artery (n=26), middle cerebral artery (n=17), and an artery in the posterior circulation (n=5).

van der Wee N, Rinkel GJ, Hasan D, van Gijn J. Detection of subarachnoid haemorrhage on early CT: is lumbar puncture still needed after a negative scan? J Neurol Neurosurg Psychiatry. 1995 Mar;58(3):357–9.

Additional Review:

Cortnum S, Sørensen P, Jørgensen J. Determining the sensitivity of computed tomography scanning in early detection of subarachnoid hemorrhage. Neurosurgery. 2010 May;66(5):900–2.

Connolly ES, Rabinstein AA, Carhuapoma JR, Derdeyn CP, Dion J, Higashida RT, et al. Guidelines for the Management of Aneurysmal Subarachnoid Hemorrhage A Guideline for Healthcare Professionals From the American Heart Association/American Stroke Association. Stroke. 2012 Jun 1;43(6):1711–37.

The Canadian CT Head Rule

1. The Canadian CT Head Rule consists of 7 predictor variables to assess the need for computed tomography (CT) imaging in patients with minor head injuries (Table I).

2. This study demonstrated that the rule is highly sensitive and may help to reduce the number of CT scans ordered.

Original Date of Publication: May 2001

Study Rundown: Minor head injury is frequently encountered in the emergency department and is defined as having a history of loss of consciousness, amnesia, or disorientation and a Glasgow Coma Scale (GCS) score of 13-15. With increasing use of head CT in this clinical scenario, conflicting guidelines emerged regarding the threshold for deciding whom to scan. In 2001, the Canadian CT Head Rule was developed with the intent of standardizing patient management while reducing the number of unnecessary scans. This landmark study developed the rule based on a large prospective cohort and found it to be a highly sensitive clinical decision tool for patients with minor head injuries, while also helping to reduce the number of unnecessary CT scans ordered.

In-Depth [prospective cohort]: This trial was carried out in 10 Canadian community and academic centers. The primary outcome was the need for neurological intervention (i.e., death within 7 days due to head injury, or need for craniotomy, elevation of skull fracture, intracranial pressure monitoring, or intubation for head injury within 7 days), while the secondary outcome was the presence of clinically important brain injury identified on CT. Patients requiring a CT were identified by standardized physician assessments, which included assessing for pre-determined predictor variables. Patients not requiring a CT were followed-up with a phone call 14 days after their assessment. A total of 3121 patients were enrolled, and 2078 of these patients received CT scans. Logistic regression was used to develop a model for identifying cases with clinically important brain injury, and the model was used to generate the 7 predictors in the Canadian CT Head Rule.

Subsequent analyses demonstrated that the 5 "high risk" factors had a sensitivity of 100% (95%CI 92-100%) and specificity of 68.7% (95%CI 67-70%) for neurological intervention, while CT scans would have been ordered in 32.2% of patients. When all 7 factors were considered, the sensitivity was 98.4% (95%CI 96-99%) and specificity was 49.6% (95%CI 48-51%) for clinically-important brain injury on CT, while CT scans would have been ordered in 54.3% of patients.

Stiell IG, Wells GA, Vandemheen K, Clement C, Lesiuk H, Laupacis A, et al. The Canadian CT Head Rule for patients with minor head injury. Lancet. 2001 May 5;357(9266):1391–6.

Canadian CT Head Rule CT head is only required for *minor head injury* patients with any of these findings:
High risk (for neurological intervention) **1.** GCS score <15 at 2 hours after injury **2.** Suspected open or depressed skull fracture **3.** Any sign of basal skull fracture (i.e., hemotympanum, "racoon" eyes, CSF otorrhea/rhinorrhea, battle's sign) **4.** Vomiting ≥2 episodes **5.** Age ≥65 years
Medium risk (for brain injury on CT) **1.** Amnesia before impact ≥30 minutes **2.** Dangerous mechanism (i.e., pedestrian struck by motor vehicle, occupant ejected from motor vehicle, fall from elevation ≥3 feet/5 stairs)

Table I. The Canadian CT Head Rule.

Canadian C-Spine Rules superior to NEXUS Low-Risk Criteria for detecting cervical-spine injuries

1. The Canadian C-Spine Rule (CCR, Figure I) demonstrated higher sensitivity and specificity for cervical-spine injury compared to the National Emergency X-Radiography Utilization Study (NEXUS) Low-Risk Criteria (NLC, Table I).

Original Date of Publication: December 2003

Study Rundown: According to large trauma registries, approximately 3% of all blunt trauma victims sustain injuries to the spinal column, including injuries to the cervical spine (C-spine). Suspected C-spine fractures are frequently evaluated with radiography; however, there is a lack of consensus among published guidelines with regards to the use of radiography. Two independently validated clinical decision rules are commonly used to determine patient selection of C-spine radiography: the CCR and the NLC. The CCR is a three-step process that evaluates risk factors for serious injury, physical exam findings, and the patient's ability to rotate their neck. The NLC is made up of five criteria based on patient history (no painful distracting injuries, normal level of consciousness) and physical examination (midline cervical tenderness, focal neurologic deficits, and no evidence of intoxication). The purpose of this landmark prospective trial was to compare the accuracy of both the CCR and the NLC in detecting C-spine injuries.

The prospective trial measured the frequency of clinically important C-spine injuries in over 8000 consecutive patients and reported the accuracy of both the CCR and NLC in detecting these injuries when applied to this cohort. At the conclusion of the trial, the CCR demonstrated a near 100% sensitivity for detecting clinically important C-spine fractures; this was significantly higher than the NLC (90.7%). Additionally, the CCR was also found to be more specific for C-spine injuries compared to NLC. When the sensitivity and specificity were applied to the cohort, the NLC would have missed 1 in 10 clinically important C-spine fractures while requiring a higher radiography rate. Ten percent (10%) of patients were not evaluated for neck range of motion and therefore did not complete the CCR algorithm. However, the sensitivity and specificity of the CCR remained significantly higher than the NLC even if all significant findings in this small subgroup were assumed to be missed by CCR.

The results of this trial demonstrated superior performance of the CCR over the NLC in detecting clinically significant C-spine injuries and supported the use of CCR as the preferred clinical prediction rule. However, the study population was only limited to patients aged greater than 16 years who were alert and in stable condition at the time of assessment. Additionally, the study was performed at institutions where the CCR was developed, precluding validation in alternative clinical settings.

In-Depth [prospective cohort]: This was a prospective study of 8282 consecutive patients with acute trauma to the head and neck for assessment for C-spine injuries in nine tertiary care hospitals in Canada. Patients were included if they were at least 16 years of age and had a Glasgow Coma Scale score of 15 out of 15 at the time of assessment. Patients were excluded if they had penetrating neck trauma, acute paralysis, or were pregnant. All patients were assessed by the CCR and NLC for the study, which was completed by the evaluating emergency physician. Patients underwent plain radiography according to the judgement of the physician independent of the results of the clinical prediction rules. All injuries to the C-spine on radiography were considered significant unless one of the following benign fractures were seen in isolation: transverse process not involving a facet joint, a spinous process not involving lamina, or simple vertebral compression of <25% of body height. Patients who did not receive radiography were evaluated for C-spine injuries using the Proxy Outcome Assessment Tool, which assessed clinical symptoms 14-days following injury.

At the conclusion of the trial, a total of 169 patients (2%) demonstrated a clinically significant C-spine fracture. The sensitivity for detection of these C-spine fractures was significantly higher in the CCR compared to the NLC (99.4% versus 90.7%; $p < 0.001$). Additionally, the CCR also demonstrated significantly higher specificity for C-spine injuries compared to NLC (40.4% versus 33.0%; $p < 0.001$). In 845 patients (10.2%), the CCR assessment was indeterminate due to failure to evaluate neck range of motion. In secondary analysis, if all indeterminate cases were assumed to be negative by the CCR, the sensitivity and specificity was modified to 95.3% and 50.7%, respectively. This remained significantly higher when compared to the NLC.

Stiell IG, Clement CM, McKnight RD, Brison R, Schull MJ, Rowe BH, et al. The Canadian C-Spine Rule versus the NEXUS Low-Risk Criteria in Patients with Trauma. The New England Journal of Medicine. 2003 Dec 25;349(26):2510–8.

Nexus Low Risk Criteria
Cervical spine radiography is indicated for trauma unless the patient exhibits all of the following criteria: 1. No posterior midline cervical tenderness 2. No focal neurological deficit 3. Normal alertness 4. No intoxication 5. No painful distracting injury

Table I. Nexus Low Risk Criteria.

Canadian C-Spine Rule

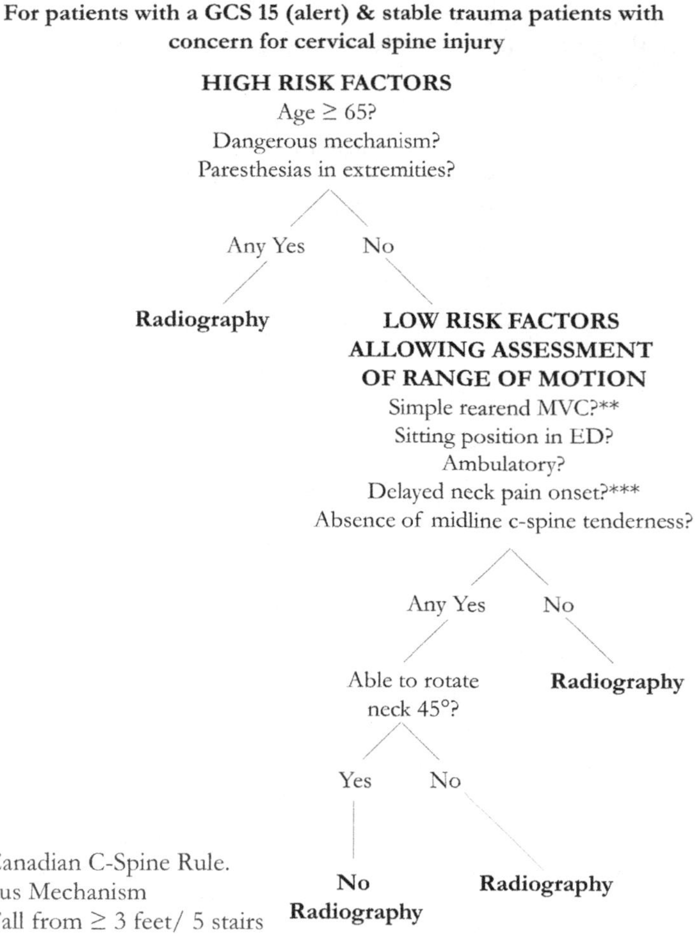

Figure I. Canadian C-Spine Rule.

* Dangerous Mechanism
- Fall from ≥ 3 feet/ 5 stairs
- Axial load to head
- High speed motor vehicle accident (MVC) ≥ 100 km/hr, rollover, ejection
- Motorized recreational vehicles
- Bicycle struck or collision

** Simple Rearend MVC Excludes
- Pushed into oncoming traffic
- Hit by bus/large truck
- Rollover
- Hit by high speed vehicle

*** Delayed
- i.e., no immediate onset of neck pain

Clinical rules accurately predict children at low risk of clinically-important traumatic brain injury

1. This validated clinical prediction tool (Figure I) accurately predicted children at a very low risk of clinically-important brain injury (ciTBI) after head trauma.

2. Two different prediction rules were developed for children over and under 2 years of age.

Original Date of Publication: September 2009

Study Rundown: Traumatic brain injuries are common within the pediatric population, resulting in over 500 000 emergency department (ED) visits annually for children under the age of 14. Computed tomography (CT) is the most commonly used imaging modality for assessment of suspected traumatic brain injuries given its widespread availability and accuracy in detecting ciTBI. However, the decision to proceed with CT for children must be balanced with the exposure to ionizing radiation in this young population, particularly in children with apparently minor head trauma. The purpose of this landmark trial was to validate and assess the accuracy of clinical prediction rules to identify children with very low risk ciTBI, who can avoid undergoing a routine CT scan.

The study prospectively analyzed the clinical outcomes of over 42 000 children who presented to the ED with a minor head trauma and a Glasgow Coma Scale (GCS) of 14 to 15. From the derivation cohort, two clinical prediction rules were created for children younger and older than 2 years of age. These prediction rules were validated with a cohort of over 8000 cases of pediatric head trauma. At the conclusion of the trial, for patients younger than two years of age, the clinical prediction tool correctly identified all patients who met the low-risk criteria for ciTBI with a sensitivity and negative predictive value for ciTBI of 100%. For patients older than 2 years of age, the clinical prediction tool demonstrated similar performance with a sensitivity and negative predictive value of 96.8% and 99.9%, respectively, for patients that meet the very low-risk criteria to require neuroimaging. This trial is strengthened by the large sample size and the use of diverse pediatric populations. To date, it is the only clinical prediction tool to be prospectively validated. These clinical prediction rules may help to identify a large group of children presenting with head trauma who meet low-risk criteria for neuroimaging an in whom CT scan could be avoided.

In-Depth [prospective cohort]: This was a prospective observational trial of 42 412 children who presented with a complaint of head trauma across 25 EDs in North America. Key exclusion criteria included known penetrating trauma, neurological disorder, or GCS less than 14 at time of presentation. The primary outcome of interest was the rate of ciTBI, defined as death from traumatic brain injury, neurosurgery, intubation for traumatic brain injury, or hospital admission of two nights or more associated with traumatic brain injury. Outcomes for discharged patients were followed up by standardized telephone surveys of parents between 7 and 90 days after ED discharge. Two clinical prediction rules were created from a derivation cohort of 33 875 children. The prediction tool for patients less than 2 years of age included normal mental status, no scalp hematoma except frontal, loss of consciousness for less than 5 seconds, non-severe injury mechanism, no palpable skull fracture, and normal behavior. The prediction tool for patients 2 years of age or older included normal mental status, no loss of consciousness, no vomiting, non-severe injury mechanism, no signs of basilar skull fracture and no severe headache. Patients with altered mental status and signs of fracture were deemed to meet high-risk criteria. Patients meeting criteria other than altered mental status or signs of fracture were considered to be intermediate-risk. Using a validation cohort of 8627 children, the prediction rule for patients younger than 2 years demonstrated a negative predictive value for ciTBI of 100% (95%CI 99.7 to 100%) and sensitivity of 100% (95%CI 86.3 to 100%). The prediction rule for patients older than 2 years of age demonstrated a negative predictive value for ciTBI of 99.9% (95%CI 99.8 to 99.99%) and a sensitivity of 96.8% (95%CI 89 to 99.6%). Patients meeting high risk criteria are recommended to undergo neuroimaging. Patients meeting intermediate risk criteria should be considered for neuroimaging incorporating clinician experience and parental comfort into the decision making process.

Kuppermann N, Holmes JF, Dayan PS, Hoyle JD, Atabaki SM, Holubkov R, et al. Identification of children at very low risk of clinically-important brain injuries after head trauma: a prospective cohort. The Lancet. 2009 Oct;374(9696):1160–70.

Child < 2 Years Old

GCS = 14?
Signs of Altered Mental Status?
Palpable Skull Fracture?

Any Yes → **CT Recommended**

No → Occipital, parietal, temporal scalp hematoma?
LOC ≥ 5s
Severe mechanism of injury?
Not acting normally per parent?

- *Any Yes* → **CT vs. Observation**
- *No* → **No CT**

Child ≥ 2 Years Old

GCS = 14?
Signs of Altered Mental Status?
Palpable Skull Fracture?

Any Yes → **CT Recommended**

No → LOC?
Vomiting?
Severe mechanism of injury?
Severe headache?

- *Any Yes* → **CT vs. Observation**
- *No* → **No CT**

Figure I. Prediction Tool Algorithm. GCS = Glasgow Coma Scale; LOC = Loss of Consciousness.

Diffusion-weighted MRI highly sensitive for acute stroke

1. Among patients with acute neurologic deficits presenting within 6 hours of symptom onset, diffusion-weighted magnetic resonance imaging (DWI) was significantly more sensitive and specific for the diagnosis of ischemic stroke compared with non-contrast computed tomography (NCCT).

Original Date of Publication: September 2002

Study Rundown: Intravenous thrombolysis is a widely accepted method for the management of acute ischemic stroke, with the goal of opening blocked vessels to restore blood flow to at-risk brain tissue. One of the primary requirements for the administration of intravenous thrombolytic drugs is the exclusion of intracranial hemorrhage as an explanation for a patient's acute neurologic symptoms. NCCT is the method of choice for fast and accurate detection of intracranial bleeding. Its performance in the detection of early acute ischemic stroke, however, is generally poor, with a reported sensitivity of approximately 40-60% within the first 6 hours from symptom onset. DWI is an imaging technique that allows for sensitive detection of ischemic stroke much earlier than is possible with NCCT.

In this comparative trial, patients presenting to the emergency department with symptoms concerning for acute ischemic stroke were assigned to undergo both NCCT and DWI in a randomized order. For each patient and for each imaging study, the presence or absence of stroke was determined alongside other parameters to determine the diagnostic utility of both methods. The results suggested that DWI is significantly more sensitive and specific than NCCT for the diagnosis of acute ischemic stroke. Additionally, researchers found that inter-reader reliability differed substantially between the two imaging modalities, with almost perfect agreement when using DWI and only modest agreement when using NCCT, suggesting that DWI is less susceptible to interpretive errors than NCCT. This was the first trial to provide a head-to-head comparison of the two diagnostic imaging methods for stroke, and it served to significantly strengthen the evidence in support of DWI, building on the results of prior trials.

In-Depth [prospective cohort]: In this study, 54 consecutive patients presenting to a single academic medical center emergency department with symptoms concerning for acute ischemic stroke were prospectively enrolled to undergo both NCCT and DWI in a randomized order. Primary inclusion criteria included presentation for evaluation within six hours of symptom onset and a National Institute of Health Stroke Scale (NIHSS) greater than 3, with higher values indicating greater stroke severity. All images were read by expert neuroradiologists and stroke neurologists and categorized according to the presence or absence of ischemic stroke, the vascular distribution of the stroke, the stroke subtype (none, lacunar, territorial, or hemodynamic), and other parameters. Readers were blinded to the specific details of each case.

Overall, NCCT demonstrated a sensitivity and specificity of 61% and 65%, respectively, for the diagnosis of acute ischemic stroke, and inter-reader reliability was moderate. DWI significantly outperformed NCCT, with a sensitivity and specificity of 91% and 95%, respectively, and almost perfect inter-reader reliability. Notably, no acute lacunar infarcts were visible on NCCT while four were diagnosed using DWI, suggesting that DWI may also be superior for the identification of specific stroke subtypes. All infarcts in this study were within the middle cerebral artery distribution, and the mean NIHSS of enrolled patients was 11 (range 3-27). The mean time from initial evaluation to the performance of diagnostic imaging was comparable for both modalities (NCCT = 180 minutes, DWI = 189 minutes).

Fiebach JB, Schellinger PD, Jansen O, Meyer M, Wilde P, Bender J, et al. CT and Diffusion-Weighted MR Imaging in Randomized Order: Diffusion-Weighted Imaging Results in Higher Accuracy and Lower Interrater Variability in the Diagnosis of Hyperacute Ischemic. Stroke. 2002 Sep 1;33(9):2206–10.

Thrombolysis harmful in acute ischemic strokes with a large area of parenchymal hypoattenuation

1. Parenchymal hypoattenuation of greater than 33% of the middle cerebral artery (MCA) territory on computed tomographic (CT) imaging within 6 hours of onset of an acute stroke was predictive of poor neurologic outcomes with intravenous thrombolytic therapy (t-PA) and an increased risk of hemorrhagic conversion.

2. Like those with a large area of focal hypoattenuation, patients without parenchymal abnormalities on CT showed a significantly increased risk of cerebral hemorrhage and no significant change in neurologic outcomes at 90-days post-t-PA; however, those with small (<33% of MCA territory) regions of hypoattenuation showed a significant improvement in long-term function.

Original Date of Publication: November 1997

Study Rundown: Acute ischemic stroke occurs when blood supply to a region of the brain is disrupted, leading to characteristic symptomatology related to the location of the lesion. After clinical examination, the mainstay of stroke diagnostics depends upon neuroimaging to aid in lesion localization and characterization of its type, size, and the extent of irreversible ischemia to guide therapeutic intervention. While recent trials have established mechanical thrombectomy as the optimal therapeutic strategy in large-vessel occlusions, the initial management of ischemic strokes presenting within 3-6 hours of onset was previously established by the ECASS and NINDS trials (Section *IV. Interface Literature*), which revealed that early t-PA administration may achieve chemical recanalization and improve neurologic recovery. The success of both newer intraarterial therapies and standard intravenous t-PA administration relies on the presence of a region of hypoperfused or "penumbral" tissue within the affected vascular territory that may be rescued by the restoration of blood flow. The referenced study sought to determine if a large area of hypoattenuation on initial CT, indicative of irreversible ischemic infarct, may portend poorer outcomes with standard t-PA treatment. Patients presenting with acute ischemic stroke within 6 hours of symptom onset underwent baseline head CT and were randomized to receive either t-PA or placebo. Patients were then prospectively subcategorized into one of three groups according to the extent of visible MCA territorial hypoattenuation: no visible defects, 33% or less, or more than 33% of the region affected, and neurologic outcomes were recorded at 90 days post-treatment. The authors found that those with greater than 33% of the MCA territory visibly hypoattenuated and those with no visible hypoattenuation on initial CT imaging did not have a statistically significant improvement in long-term neurologic recovery, but did suffer a significantly increased risk of fatal cerebral hemorrhage secondary to t-PA therapy. Those with hypoattenuation visible in less than 33% of the MCA territory were not at significantly increased risk of hemorrhagic conversion and demonstrated an improvement in long-term neurologic recovery, as observed in the previously referenced trials. This analysis was instrumental in demonstrating that the extent of completed ischemia visible on CT could predict outcomes after stroke therapy.

In-Depth [randomized controlled trial]: A total of 620 patients presenting with acute, ischemic hemispheric stroke within 6 hours of symptom onset were randomized to either receive intravenous t-PA or placebo in a double-blinded fashion across multiple European medical centers. All patients underwent baseline head CT, and were prospectively categorized into one of three groups according to the extent of hypoattenuation visible within the affected MCA territory: no hypoattenuation visible, less than 33% (small territory), or greater than 33% (large territory). Of those enrolled, 336 patients had no visible parenchymal hypoattenuation, while 215 displayed a small region, and only 52 displayed a large region of hypoattenuation, and no significant differences in baseline characteristics were noted between the subcategories except for their presenting clinical stroke scores (progressively worsened for those with larger areas of infarction; $p < 0.0001$). The degree of presenting hypoattenuation was significantly associated with an increased baseline risk of poor neurologic outcomes as assessed within the placebo-treated groups ($p < 0.0001$). Among patients treated with intravenous t-PA, no statistically significant effect on long-term neurologic recovery was noted for patients with either no initial parenchymal hypoattenuation or those with a large area of parenchymal hypoattenuation. However, 14 of 198 patients (7%) in these two groups died secondary to cerebral hemorrhage, while only 2 of 190 patients (1%) in the corresponding placebo-treated groups suffered the same complication. Patients who presented with a small area of hypoattenuation displayed an OR for good neurologic recovery of 3.43 following t-PA treatment, while those with a large or no area of hypoattenuation did not show a significant difference in their odds of recovery (OR 0.41, 95%CI 0.06-2.70; OR 1.27, 95%CI 0.82-1.95, respectively). This study established the lack of benefit and subsequent risks of utilizing intravenous thrombolytic therapy in patients with greater than one-third of the MCA territory visibly infarcted.

Von Kummer R, Allen KL, Holle R, Bozzao L, Bastianello S, Manelfe C, et al. Acute stroke: Usefulness of early CT findings before thrombolytic therapy. Radiology. *1997 Nov 1;205(2):327–33.*

Hacke W, Kaste M, Fieschi C, Toni D, Lesaffre E, Kummer R von, et al. Intravenous Thrombolysis With Recombinant Tissue Plasminogen Activator for Acute Hemispheric Stroke: The European Cooperative Acute Stroke Study (ECASS). JAMA. 1995 Oct 4;274(13):1017–25.

The National Institute of Neurological Disorders and Stroke rt-PA Stroke Study Group. Tissue plasminogen activator for acute ischemic stroke. The New England Journal of Medicine. 1995 Dec 14;333(24):1581–87.

Medical management superior to stenting for stroke related to intracranial arterial stenosis

1. The risk of early stroke after angioplasty and stenting of intracranial atherosclerotic lesions was higher than expected, while the risk of stroke with aggressive medical therapy alone was lower than expected.

2. The probability of ischemic stroke, symptomatic brain hemorrhage, and non-stroke related death after stenting plus medical management was significantly greater than medical management alone.

Original Date of Publication: September 2011

Study Rundown: Atherosclerotic intracranial arterial stenosis is an important cause of ischemic stroke and a major predictor of recurrent stroke following an initial event. Antiplatelet therapy and risk factor management have long been regarded as mainstays in the treatment and prevention of recurrent stroke. However, with the approval of the first self-expanding nitinol stent by the Food and Drug Administration (FDA) in 2005 for use in patients with atherosclerotic intracranial arterial stenosis, percutaneous transluminal angioplasty and stenting (PTAS) in addition to antithrombotic therapy emerged as a potential alternative approach towards the treatment of high-risk patients.

In the randomized controlled trial conducted by Chimowitz and colleagues, the safety and efficacy of PTAS and medical therapy was compared to medical therapy alone in high-risk patients with intracranial arterial stenosis. The results of this trial showed that aggressive medical management alone was superior to PTAS plus medical management, demonstrating a lower risk of recurrent ischemic stroke.

In-Depth [randomized controlled trial]: This study was conducted in 50 sites across the United States. To be considered eligible for participation in the study, patients must have experienced a transient ischemic attack (TIA) or nondisabling stroke within 30 days of enrollment, attributed to intracranial arterial stenosis of 70-99% of a major intracranial artery. Arterial stenosis was verified angiographically. Patients with tandem extracranial or intracranial stenosis, an occlusion located proximally or distally to the target intracranial lesion, or bilateral intracranial vertebral artery stenosis were excluded.

Following screening and consent, patients were randomized to receive PTAS and medical management or medical management alone. Medical therapy consisted of 325 mg of aspirin and 75 mg of clopidogrel, both administered daily for 90 days after enrollment, as well as management of primary (elevated systolic blood pressure and low-density lipoprotein (LDL) cholesterol levels) and secondary risk factors (diabetes, elevated non-high-density lipoprotein (non-HDL) cholesterol levels, smoking, excess weight and sedentarism) through a lifestyle modification program. Primary endpoints of the study included ischemic stroke, symptomatic brain hemorrhage, and non-stroke related death within 30 days after enrollment, as well as ischemic stroke in the territory of the qualifying lesion beyond 30 days of enrollment.

A total of 451 patients were randomized to receive either PTAS and medical therapy (n=224; mean age 61.0 years, SD 10.7; 56.7% male) or medical therapy alone (n=227; mean age 59.5 years, SD 11.8 years; 63.9% male). There were no significant differences between the groups with respect to baseline patient characteristics. In the PTAS group, the probability of experiencing any primary end point within 30 days after enrollment was considerably higher at 14.7% compared to 5.8% in the medical management group ($p = 0.002$). In addition, while no patients in the medical management group experienced symptomatic brain hemorrhage during the 30-day follow-up period, 10 of the 33 strokes (30.3%) in the PTAS group resulted in this outcome ($p = 0.04$). Over 1 year of follow-up, the probability of experiencing a primary endpoint was also significantly greater in the PTAS group (20.2%) compared to the medical management group (12.2%, $p = 0.009$).

Chimowitz MI, Lynn MJ, Derdeyn CP, Turan TN, Fiorella D, Lane BF, et al. Stenting versus aggressive medical therapy for intracranial arterial stenosis. The New England Journal of Medicine. 2011 Sep;365(11):993-1003.

Middle cerebral artery doppler velocimetry predicts fetal anemia

1. Among fetuses at risk for maternal red cell alloimmunization, peak systolic velocity in the middle cerebral artery (MCA) was a sensitive predictor of moderate or severe fetal anemia.

Original Date of Publication: January 2000

Study Rundown: Maternal red cell alloimmunization is a morbid immunogenic phenomenon associated with a high risk of fetal anemia that complicates less than 1% of pregnancies. Maternal alloimmunization results when a pregnant woman previously sensitized to a paternally-derived red cell antigen is re-exposed by a fetus that carries the same paternally-derived antigen. In response, maternal antibodies are produced, cross the placenta, bind to antigens on fetal red blood cells, and cause hemolysis. In severe cases, hemolysis can progress to severe fetal anemia, hydrops fetalis, and fetal death. As of the late 1990s, women at risk for alloimmunization underwent invasive testing via serial cordocentesis, the standard of care, or amniocenteses to diagnose fetal anemia. Cordocentesis permitted direct measurement of fetal hemoglobin, but exposed women to a 1-2% risk of fetal loss and a 50% risk of fetal-maternal hemorrhage, which worsens alloimmunization. Amniocentesis carried less risk, but was unreliable at diagnosis anemia due to the wide variation in bilirubin levels in amniotic fluid. Researchers hypothesized that measuring peak systolic velocity in a fetal cerebral artery might permit reliable yet noninvasive anemia diagnosis. A prior study demonstrated that peak systolic velocity through the fetal MCA, as measured by ultrasound, was increased in anemic infants. In this study, researchers compared measurement of peak systolic middle cerebral artery velocimetry to the current standard of care, invasive cordocentesis, for diagnosis of fetal anemia among infants at risk for maternal alloimmunization.

This landmark study demonstrated that increased peak systolic velocity through the fetal middle cerebral artery is a sensitive predictor of moderate or severe fetal anemia. Findings allowed for noninvasive diagnosis of fetal anemia and prevent fetuses with mild anemia from exposure to the morbidity and mortality associated with invasive testing. Authors calculated that institution of doppler velocimetry for screening and diagnosis of fetal anemia would prevent an estimated 140 pregnancy losses associated with cordocentesis each year. Strengths included the multicenter study design, concomitant measurement of hemoglobin by both direct (cordocentesis) and indirect (doppler velocimetry) methods, and use of a control population. Limitations included small sample size to evaluate variation in velocity associated with diagnosis of the rare, fatal outcome of fetal hydrops (n=11).

In-Depth [cross-sectional study]: A total of 111 fetuses at risk for anemia due to maternal red cell alloimmunization underwent measurement of hemoglobin concentration via invasive cordocentesis and via noninvasive measurement of MCA peak systolic velocity using doppler velocimetry. Hemoglobin values in at-risk infants were compared to the hemoglobin values of 265 normal fetuses in this comparative cross-sectional study. The outcome of interest was moderate fetal anemia, defined as hemoglobin <0.65 times the median hemoglobin concentration in normal fetuses and severe anemia, defined as <0.55 times the median.

Peak MCA systolic velocity values greater than 1.5 times the median conferred 100% sensitivity and a 100% negative predictive value for the diagnosis of moderate or severe fetal anemia. The relationship between multiples of the median of peak systolic velocity with moderate to severe fetal anemia was significant ($p < 0.001$). Among infants at risk for anemia related to maternal alloimmunization, 32% had mild anemia, 4% had moderate anemia and 28% had severe anemia.

Mari G, Deter RL, Carpenter RL, Rahman F, Zimmerman R, Moise KJ, Jr., et al. Noninvasive diagnosis by Doppler ultrasonography of fetal anemia due to maternal red-cell alloimmunization. Collaborative Group for Doppler Assessment of the Blood Velocity in Anemic Fetuses. The New England Journal of Medicine. 2000;342(1):9-14.

MRI reveals lumbar intervertebral disk herniations are common in asymptomatic individuals

1. Magnetic resonance imaging (MRI) of the lumbar spine in individuals without back pain revealed that at least a single intervertebral disk bulge was prevalent in over half of those imaged, while over a quarter showed at least a single disk protrusion.

2. Other abnormalities were common, including Schmorl's nodes, defects of the annulus fibrosis, and facet arthropathy, without significant differences in the prevalence of any given abnormality between the sexes.

Original Date of Publication: July 1994

Study Rundown: Low back pain remains a difficult management dilemma given the chronicity of most complaints and poor symptomatic response to intervention, leading to a great deal of unnecessary spinal imaging at significant cost to the medical system. Even in light of positive findings on imaging, clinicians have had difficulty correlating symptoms to imaging findings. Prior to this study, "herniation" was an amorphous term used to describe the spectrum of intervertebral disk abnormalities seen on MRI ranging from small bulges, to larger protrusions or even complete extrusions. The authors of this study showed that among individuals without back pain, the prevalence of at least a single disk bulge was 52% on MRI of the lumbar spine, with an age-dependent association demonstrated for both the number of disks affected and the prevalence of bulges seen. Disk protrusions were evident in 27% of asymptomatic individuals, while extrusions were found in only 1% of those imaged. The vast majority of disk abnormalities were found at the L4-5 and L5-S1 spaces, and least commonly at the L1-2 space. Similarly, findings of Schmorl's nodes, or disk herniation into an adjacent vertebral body end plate, annular defects, and facet arthropathy were seen in 19%, 14%, and 8% of asymptomatic subjects, respectively. These findings, in light of the more specific terminology introduced, demonstrated that disk bulges and protrusions, but not extrusions, were highly prevalent in the population and could not reliably predict symptoms of back pain, and in fact may be purely coincidental.

In-Depth [prospective cohort]: This prospective trial enrolled 98 volunteers without back pain symptoms (mean age 42.3 years; 49% female) at a community hospital in California. Exclusion criteria included a history of back pain lasting greater than 48 hours or any history of lumbosacral radiculopathies. Each subject underwent 1.5T MRI of the lumbar spine in both the axial and sagittal planes, and completed a survey to score their level of baseline physical activity from 0 (no exercise) to 4 (five or more workouts per week). In addition to the 98 MRIs produced for these subjects, 27 abnormal studies of the lumbar spine were randomly intermixed to reduce interpretation bias. All studies were interpreted independently by a pair of experienced neuroradiologists at an outside academic medical center blinded to the clinical status of the study subjects, and results of the two readings were averaged for final summary of the data. The specific nomenclature used to describe intervertebral disk findings was described as follows: Normal (without disk extension beyond the interspace), bulge (with symmetric extension of the disk beyond the interspace), protrusion (with asymmetric extension of the disk beyond the interspace), or extrusion (with the extruding disk material larger in diameter than the remaining disk in the interspace).

Among the asymptomatic individuals imaged, 52% had a disk bulge at at least one level, 27% demonstrated at least one protrusion, and only 1% demonstrated an extrusion, for a total of 64% of those without back pain demonstrating a disk abnormality at one level and 38% with abnormalities at more than one level. Abnormalities of the intervertebral disks were most prevalent at the L5-S1 and L4-5 levels, with a decreasing prevalence toward the L1-2 level. There were no differences in the prevalence of disk abnormalities between the sexes, but an increase in the prevalence of disk bulges was seen with increasing age ($p < 0.001$) at every disk level. Age also predicted an increase in the prevalence of multiple disk abnormalities ($p < 0.001$). The physical activity score did not correlate significantly to the number of visualized disk abnormalities. A variety of other, non-intervertebral disk spinal abnormalities were noted among those imaged: Most commonly, Schmorl's nodes were noted in 19% of subjects, defects of the annulus fibrosis in 14%, facet arthropathy in 8%, and spondylolysis, spondylolisthesis, central canal stenosis, and neural foraminal stenosis were each seen in 7% of imaged subjects.

Jensen MC, Brant-Zawadzki MN, Obuchowski N, Modic MT, Malkasian D, Ross JS. Magnetic Resonance Imaging of the Lumbar Spine in People Without Back Pain. The New England Journal of Medicine. 1994 Jul 14;331(2):69–73.

Ottawa ankle rules reduce the rate of referral for ankle radiography

1. The Ottawa ankle rules significantly reduced referral for ankle, but not foot, radiography in the emergency department.

2. Patients without fractures spent less time in the emergency department if not referred for radiography without an increased rate of missed fractures.

Original Date of Publication: September 1995

Study Rundown: Ankle and foot injuries are some of the most common complaints evaluated in the emergency department. While relatively few patients sustain a fracture related to their injury, it has long been standard practice to perform plain radiography of the ankle and/or foot on virtually all patients. This, along with unreliable findings made through history taking and physical examination defined the need for decision rules on the use of radiography for acute ankle injuries. The Ottawa ankle rules (Table I) were designed to allow physicians to rapidly identify patients with a negligible risk of fracture based on the assessment of weight-bearing ability and areas of bone tenderness. These decision rules have subsequently been validated and are highly sensitive in identifying fractures.

In the large multicenter trial conducted by Stiell and colleagues, rates of referral for ankle and foot injuries were compared before and after the introduction of the Ottawa ankle rules. The results of this study showed that implementation of the Ottawa ankle rules significantly reduced referral for ankle radiography. Patients without fractures also spent less time in the emergency department if they were not referred for radiography without an increased rate of missed fractures.

In-Depth [non-randomized controlled trial]: This study was conducted across 8 emergency departments in Canada. All adult patients seen at a participating study site with an ankle injury during the 12-month control (before) or intervention (after) periods were included. Before the start of the intervention period, the Ottawa ankle rules were introduced by means of a 1 hour lecture and supported by handouts, pocket cards and posters in each emergency department. The decision to order radiography was left to the discretion of the treating physician. Treating physicians included emergency and family physicians as well as housestaff. Referral for radiography was determined through radiology reports. As part of the intervention, patients deemed to be without fracture were followed up by telephone after 10 days if they did not receive any radiography. Patients that were seen during the first 7 days of each month and received radiography were also followed up.

A total of 12 777 eligible patients (median age 32, range 18-101; 53% men) were seen in a participating emergency department for treatment of an ankle injury. Patients evaluated during the pre-intervention (n=6288) and intervention (n=6489) periods did not significantly differ with respect to any baseline patient characteristics. During the pre-intervention period, 82.8% of patients were referred for ankle radiography compared to 60.9% during the intervention period ($p < 0.001$), corresponding to a relative reduction of 26.4%. For 4.9% of cases, radiography was unnecessarily performed according to the Ottawa ankle rules, where only 0.5% of these cases were the result of patient insistence. The proportion of patients referred for ankle imaging was significantly less at all 8 participating hospitals and across all physician subgroups. For foot imaging, however, significant reductions in referral were noted at only 3 of the 8 study sites. Among patients without fracture, those that were not referred for radiography spent less time in the emergency department compared to patients that underwent imaging studies ($p < 0.001$). Of the 2033 patients comprising the follow up group, 10 (0.5%) had a fracture diagnosed after discharge despite no repeat injury, 7 of which had not received radiography (n=1301). It should be noted, however, that the Ottawa ankle rules were correctly applied in only 1 of the 7 patients from the latter follow-up group. A cost minimization analysis also showed that the mean total expense for patients who had no radiography was less than those who had radiography ($p < 0.001$).

Stiell I, Wells G, Laupacis A, Brison R, Verbeek R, Vandemheen K, et al. Multicentre trial to introduce the Ottawa ankle rules for use of radiography in acute ankle injuries. BMJ. 1995 Sep;311(7005):594-7.

ANKLE series required if:	FOOT series required if:
1) Bone tenderness at posterior edge or tip of lateral malleolus **OR** 2) Bone tenderness at posterior edge or tip or medial malleolus **OR** 3) Inability to bear weight both immediately and in emergency department	1) Bone tenderness at base of 5th metatarsal **OR** 2) Bone tenderness at navicular **OR** 3) Inability to bear weight both immediately and in emergency department

Table I. Ottawa ankle rules.

CT evaluation in pancreatitis strongly correlates with patient outcomes

1. Among patients with acute pancreatitis, the presence and degree of pancreatic necrosis correlated with average hospital length of stay, complications, and mortality.

2. By combining an existing acute pancreatitis grading system with computed tomography (CT) evaluation of pancreatic necrosis, the authors generated a CT Severity Index that strongly correlated with patient outcomes.

Original Date of Publication: February 1990

Study Rundown: Acute pancreatitis is a common condition involving inflammation of the pancreas. Though most patients have a benign course without associated complications, some develop severe disease associated with high rates of morbidity and mortality. Numerous attempts have been made to estimate patient prognosis in acute pancreatitis, including attempts to correlate imaging findings with patient outcomes using CT. Due to limitations in early CT technology, however, pancreatitis grading scales suffered from poor sensitivity and specificity and were not widely used. In this trial, the study authors attempted to build on these prior works by using contrast-enhanced CT to evaluate the presence and degree of pancreatic necrosis as a prognostic indicator in acute pancreatitis. Using a prospective patient cohort at a single institution, the study authors demonstrated a strong, positive relationship between pancreatic necrosis and patient outcomes. Compared to those with a normal-appearing pancreas by CT, patients with necrosis had significantly longer hospital lengths of stay and higher rates of complications. All deaths in the study cohort were in patients with pancreatic necrosis. Combining this information with previously described rating scales, the authors were then able to generate the CT Severity Index (CTSI), a numeric scale to predict the risk of complications and death. Applying this scale to the study cohort, morbidity and mortality strongly correlated with CTSI score. Primary limitations of this study included modest sample size and the associated low mortality rate. Subsequent work in pancreatitis imaging has expanded upon this landmark trial and has been incorporated into a modified CTSI.

In-Depth [prospective cohort]: Eighty-eight patients (mean age, 52 years) with signs and symptoms of acute pancreatitis were enrolled. All patients were initially managed with standard medical therapy, including nasogastric suction, analgesia, and intravenous fluids. Surgical intervention was pursued in patients with sepsis refractory to medical management. All patients underwent CT imaging of the abdomen with intravenous and oral contrast for evaluation of pancreatic necrosis at the time of admission, and a subset of patients received additional, subsequent CT imaging (mean number of CTs/patients, 2.9). Scans were interpreted blindly and assessed for two specific features: the patient's five-point pancreatitis grade, based on previously published data; and the qualitative degree of decreased pancreatic parenchymal enhancement. This latter variable was taken to represent the presence of pancreatic necrosis, and was reported as one of four possible severities. Additional collected data included Ranson's score, hospital length of stay, morbidity—defined as pancreatic abscess or pseudocyst formation—and mortality.

At the end of the trial, 66 (75.0%) patients had uncomplicated courses and recovered with medical therapy alone, while 22 (25.0%) patients required surgical intervention. Five (5.7%) patients died. In total, pancreatic necrosis was detected in 18 (20.5%) patients. Average length of stay was 109 days among patients with >50% necrosis, as compared to 25 days among those without evidence of necrosis at presentation. The average Ranson's score (a marker of severity, maximum score 11) was 1.9 among those without necrosis and 5.5 among those with >50% necrosis. Patients with CT evidence of necrosis had morbidity and mortality rates of 82% and 23%, respectively, as compared with respective rates of 6% and 0% among those without necrosis. The positive predictive value for abscess formation was 77% among patients with necrosis, and the negative predictive value of abscess formation among those without necrosis was 97%. By combining pancreatitis grade and CT extent of pancreatic necrosis, a CT Severity Index was created with a maximum score of 10 (highest severity). Among study patients with a CTSI of 0-3, there was 3% mortality and 8% morbidity; among patients with a CTSI of 7-10, mortality and morbidity were 17% and 92%, respectively.

Balthazar EJ, Robinson DL, Megibow AJ, Ranson JH. Acute pancreatitis: value of CT in establishing prognosis. Radiology. 1990 Feb 1;174(2):331–6.

Magnetic resonance cholangiopancreatography diagnoses bile duct obstruction with high sensitivity and specificity

1. Magnetic resonance cholangiopancreatography (MRCP) diagnosed bile duct obstruction with high sensitivity and specificity when compared to invasive endoscopic retrograde cholangiopancreatography (ERCP).

2. MRCP was highly specific but less sensitive in identifying causes of bile duct obstruction such as malignancy or choledocholithiasis.

Original Date of Publication: October 1995

Study Rundown: Ultrasound and computed tomography have long been used in the noninvasive diagnosis of biliary obstruction, though are limited by their low sensitivity in detecting common bile duct (CBD) stones. ERCP involves endoscopically accessing the pancreatic ducts and biliary tree and directly visualizing them via injection of iodinated contrast, allowing sensitive detection of stones and other pathology as well as the capability for direct therapeutic intervention if necessary. Its invasive nature, however, remains a limitation. MRCP was created to allow noninvasive evaluation of the biliary tree using magnetic resonance imaging.

In this study conducted by Guibaud and colleagues, MRCP was compared to ERCP in the diagnosis of bile duct obstruction. The results of this study demonstrated that MRCP can be used in diagnosing bile duct obstruction with high specificity and sensitivity, with few false negative results. MRCP was also able to correctly identify choledocholithiasis or malignancy as causes of obstruction with high specificity and acceptable sensitivity, informing its subsequent increasing use as a reliable noninvasive tool in the workup of biliary obstruction.

In-Depth [prospective cohort]: All patients with clinically suspected bile duct obstruction were referred for evaluation and consecutively screened for enrollment (n=206). Patients were excluded if direct cholangiographic, histopathological or surgical proof of bile duct obstruction could not be obtained, ERCP was unsuccessful, MRCP could not be performed due to claustrophobia, or if the results of either technique were inadequate. All patients included in the study underwent MRCP with heavily T2-weighted fast spin-echo sequences. All MR images were evaluated by 2 reviewers without knowledge of clinical parameters or results of other imaging studies. The final diagnosis and, where applicable, the cause of bile duct obstruction, was determined through ERCP. The following diagnoses were considered causes of obstruction: CBD stones, malignant obstruction, chronic pancreatitis, intrahepatic stones and distal obstruction from an undetermined cause.

ERCP and MRCP were successfully performed in a total of 126 patients (mean age 57 years, range 12-91 years; 40% male). Based on the reference standard, 79 patients (63%) were found to have bile duct obstruction. Among these patients, MRCP correctly diagnosed bile duct obstruction in 72 patients, yielding a sensitivity of 91% (95%CI 85-100%) and specificity of 100%. In addition, MRCP correctly diagnosed malignancy as a cause of obstruction in 12 out of 14 patients, corresponding to a sensitivity of 86% (95%CI 67-100%) and specificity of 98% (95%CI 96-100%). In diagnosing choledocholithiasis as a cause of obstruction, the sensitivity of MRCP was less at 81% (95%CI 68-95%), with a specificity of 98% (95%CI 95-100%).

Guibaud L, Bret PM, Reinhold C, Atri M, Barkun AN. Bile duct obstruction and choledocholithiasis: diagnosis with MR cholangiography. Radiology. 1995 Oct;197(1):109-15.

Ultrasound sensitive for appendicitis, improves outcomes

1. Among patients with signs and symptoms consistent with acute appendicitis (AA), ultrasound demonstrated a sensitivity and specificity of 80% and 100%, respectively.

2. The use of ultrasound led to an appropriate change in patient management in 26.1% of cases.

Original Date of Publication: September 1987

Study Rundown: AA is a common cause of abdominal pain in both children and adults, and can be challenging to diagnose by physical examination alone. By the mid-1980s a number of small, retrospective studies had been performed suggesting a diagnostic role for graded-compression ultrasound (GCUS), a technique that involves the application of pressure to abdominal wall with the ultrasound probe to minimize obscuration by bowel gas. However, the results were felt to be equivocal, and GCUS was not widely adopted. In the present trial, the question of GCUS as a diagnostic tool in the evaluation of patients with suspected AA was addressed prospectively in a large cohort of patients at a single academic medical center. All enrolled patients were imaged after initial assessment by a surgeon, and changes in planned patient management were recorded alongside the diagnostic performance of GCUS. Results showed a high sensitivity and specificity for AA as well as a favorable trend toward improved patient care, with changes in management made for over one-quarter of patients. Notably, GCUS was not able to visualize the appendix in a significant minority of cases, in part reflecting limitations in ultrasound technology at the time of the study's publication.

In-Depth [prospective cohort]: A total of 111 consecutive patients (mean age 29 years, range 8-86 years) with a clinical presentation concerning for AA were prospectively enrolled at a single academic medical center over a 5 month period. All enrolled patients were first clinically evaluated by a member of the surgical staff using a combination of physical examination, laboratory studies, and plain x-ray images. Immediately following this, patients then received comprehensive abdominal ultrasound using graded compression for optimization of bowel visualization. All ultrasound studies were performed by radiologists and evaluated on several parameters, including appendiceal visualization, certainty of appendiceal visualization, and the presence imaging findings consistent with complications such as appendiceal perforation. After a maximum period of 6 hours of patient observation and prior to being informed of ultrasound findings, the evaluating surgeon was then asked to provide recommendations for operative or non-operative management. Imaging findings were then provided alongside an opportunity to alter management plans. The final diagnosis was determined using surgical pathology, intraoperative findings, or clinical diagnosis in combination with radiology and other supporting data.

An unequivocal ultrasound diagnosis was rendered in 83 (74.8%) patients. Among these patients, the overall sensitivity and specificity for the diagnosis of AA were 80% and 100%, respectively. When considering only those patients with non-perforated AA, the sensitivity remained essentially unchanged at 80.5% but decreased to 28.5% for patients with perforated AA. This was felt to be related to obscuration of the bowel wall by free intra-abdominal fluid and difficult patient examination secondary to peritonitis. In 29 (26.1%) patients, GCUS led to an appropriate change in management, including 16 (14.4%) patients originally triaged to conservative management who instead underwent surgical intervention. Among 4 of the 28 (14.3%) patients without a definitive final diagnosis, the appendix was unequivocally visualized but the patients did not undergo surgery because of symptom resolution.

Puylaert JBCM, Rutgers PH, Lalisang RI, de Vries BC, van der Werf SDJ, Dörr JPJ, et al. A Prospective Study of Ultrasonography in the Diagnosis of Appendicitis. The New England Journal of Medicine. 1987 Sep 10;317(11):666–9.

MRI effective for the assessment of acute appendicitis in pregnancy

1. In pregnant patients with suspected acute appendicitis and equivocal abdominal ultrasound, magnetic resonance imaging (MRI) demonstrated high accuracy, sensitivity, and negative predictive value for acute appendicitis.

Original Date of Publication: March 2006

Study Rundown: Acute appendicitis is a common cause of lower abdominal pain during pregnancy, with an incidence of 1 case per 1500 pregnancies. Ultrasonography is the initial imaging modality of choice to evaluate patients with acute right lower quadrant pain in pregnancy. However, due to the anatomical changes associated with the large gravid uterus, the sensitivity and specificity of identifying the appendix on ultrasonography is significantly lower compared to the general population. In cases of an equivocal ultrasound examination, MRI may be used to assess the appendix while avoiding ionizing radiation. The purpose of this landmark retrospective cohort was to determine the accuracy of MRI in the assessment of acute appendicitis during pregnancy.

This trial retrospectively reviewed 51 consecutive pregnant patients who were clinically suspected of having acute appendicitis that underwent MRI examinations of the abdomen with oral contrast. Positive appendicitis findings included a dilated appendix with high-signal intensity luminal fluid on T2-weigted imaging or periappendiceal fat stranding. At the conclusion of the trial, MRI demonstrated positive findings in all four patients that had confirmed acute appendicitis. No cases of appendicitis were missed by MRI. Additionally, in patients with no appendicitis, MRI demonstrated an alternate diagnosis for acute abdominal pain in 25% of patients. This study was the one of the first to demonstrate the high accuracy and negative predictive value to rule-out acute appendicitis in pregnant patients and highlighted the value of MRI in detecting periappendiceal findings as well as other potential etiologies of acute abdomen pain in pregnancy. Limitations included a small sample size and the fact that cases in which the appendix could not be visualized (16% of all patients) were classified as true negatives for statistical calculations rather than indeterminate. A number of other small retrospective reviews by Cobben et al., Brichard et al., and Israel et al., have confirmed the accuracy of MRI to be able to visualize the appendix in addition to determining other potential causes of acute abdominal pain.

In-Depth [retrospective cohort]: This study reviewed 51 consecutive pregnant patients (mean age: 28.3 years; range: 15-37, mean gestational age: 19.8 weeks; range: 4-38 weeks) that underwent oral-contrast enhanced MRI imaging of the abdomen for assessment of acute appendicitis in a single institution in the United States. 94% (48/51) of patients had ultrasound prior to MRI examination. All MRI examinations were performed on a 1.5-T coil with T1- T2-, Half-Fourier single-shot fast spin echo, and transverse time-of-flight gradient echo sequences. Interpretation of a positive finding of acute appendicitis was based on the presence of a dilated (>7 mm in diameter) appendix with high signal intensity luminal fluid on T2-weight images. Positive appendicitis was also noted if periappendiceal fat stranding was observed. The primary outcome was the accuracy, sensitivity, specificity, as well as positive and negative predictive values for appendicitis. At the conclusion of the study, MRI imaging demonstrated positive findings of appendicitis in all four cases with three inconclusive cases. All four patients with positive MRI findings had pathologically or CT-confirmed acute appendicitis. The appendix could not be visualized in 8 of the remaining 47 patients (17%) without acute appendicitis. As the study classified these nonvisualized cases as negatives rather than indeterminate, this translated into a prevalence-adjusted accuracy of 94% and a sensitivity, specificity, and negative predictive value of 100%, 93.6%, and 100%, respectively. Additionally, in patients with no evidence of acute appendicitis, MRI imaging provided an additional 58 alternative diagnoses related to the patient's acute abdominal pain, including an enlarged right gonadal vein (n=11), right hydronephrosis (n=25), degenerated fibroids (n=6), and sub-chorionic hemorrhage (n=11).

Pedrosa I, Levine D, Eyvazzadeh AD, Siewert B, Ngo L, Rofsky NM. MR Imaging Evaluation of Acute Appendicitis in Pregnancy. Radiology. 2006 Mar 1;238(3):891–9.

Additional Review:

Cobben LP, Groot I, Haans L, Blickman JG, Puylaert J. MRI for Clinically Suspected Appendicitis During Pregnancy. Am J Roentgenol. 2004 Sep 1;183(3):671–5.

Birchard KR, Brown MA, Hyslop WB, Firat Z, Semelka RC. MRI of Acute Abdominal and Pelvic Pain in Pregnant Patients. Am J Roentgenol. 2005 Feb 1;184(2):452–8.

Israel GM, Malguria N, McCarthy S, Copel J, Weinreb J. MRI versus ultrasound for suspected appendicitis during pregnancy. J Magn Reson Imaging. 2008 Aug 1;28(2):428–33.

Bosniak classification system differentiates benign renal cysts from cystic carcinoma

1. The presence of calcification, septa, irregularities or thickness in cyst walls on ultrasound (US) or computed tomography (CT) can be used to identify potentially malignant lesions requiring surgery.

2. Hyperdense cysts can be considered benign without further imaging if they demonstrate a specific appearance (smooth, round, sharply marginated, and homogeneous), lack of enhancement, and size <3 cm.

Original Date of Publication: January 1986

Study Rundown: Renal cysts are a common incidental finding on imaging studies evaluating potential abdominal or pelvic pathologies. Most often, renal cysts are discovered through US or CT. While many simple or uncomplicated cysts pose minimal difficulty in diagnosis, the optimal management of complicated cystic lesions remains controversial.

Bosniak proposed an approach for managing renal cysts using US and CT imaging features. This includes a classification system for renal cysts and cystic lesions. Category I lesions include benign simple cysts of the kidney diagnosed definitively by sonography and/or CT. Category II lesions are minimally complicated cysts that are benign but have certain radiologic features (i.e., septa, minimal calcification, infection or high density). Category III lesions are complicated cystic lesions exhibiting some but not all radiologic features of malignancy, and therefore require surgical exploration. Category IV lesions are malignant.

In-Depth [review]: Bosniak provides a detailed diagnostic algorithm for classifying and managing renal cysts using imaging features (Table I). For masses first identified through urography without clear characteristics of malignancy (i.e., fat or calcification within the mass, increased tissue density, irregularity of margins, or invasion of collection system), US should be performed with results of previous imaging available for review. If the mass does not meet all criteria for a simple cyst on US, CT examination with and without intravenous contrast should be performed. Non-contrast CT scans allow determination of whether areas of increased density on contrast-enhanced is true tissue enhancement. The Bosniak classification system (Table I) was made based on the most common and pertinent radiologic features identified through US and/or CT. This includes calcification seen within a renal lesion, which should always be interpreted as a sign of possible malignancy. While the presence of calcification can be associated with malignancy, if no other suspicious features are present, a small amount of calcium in the wall or septa of a lesion may indicate a complicated cyst without malignancy (category II lesion). However, extensive calcification in the wall of the lesion warrants category III classification requiring surgical exploration to rule out malignancy. Calcification associated with an enhancing soft-tissue mass indicates malignancy (category IV) and necessitates surgical resection.

In addition, while many benign cysts have fine septa, lesions with numerous septa, irregular septal walls, septa over 1 mm in thickness, or with associated solid elements at attachment sites should be explored surgically (category III). If numerous irregular septa are present and associated with solid areas, a cystic carcinoma (category IV) can be diagnosed. Thickening or irregularity of the wall of a lesion also excludes benignity, placing such lesions in categories III or IV, depending on the severity of findings.

Bosniak also states the importance of assessing fluid density in cysts. Hyperdense renal cysts, usually containing old blood and often seen in patients with polycystic kidney disease, have a higher attenuation than surrounding renal parenchyma on non-contrast-enhanced CT scans. Following intravenous (IV) administration of contrast material, these lesions appear either isodense or hypodense when compared to the renal parenchyma, and can be considered benign if all of the following criteria are met: a) the lesion is smooth, round, sharply marginated and homogeneous, b) the lesion does not enhance with IV administration of contrast material and does not change in configuration, and c) the lesion is 3 cm or less in size. Lesions over 3 cm in size may still be benign, though US should be used to characterize it as a fluid-filled cyst. Lesions meeting all of the above criteria do not require surgical exploration or removal but should be monitored carefully through CT surveillance.

Bosniak MA. The current radiological approach to renal cysts. Radiology. 1986 Jan;158(1):1-10.

Additional Review:

Bosniak, MA. The Bosniak Renal Cyst Classification: 25 Years Later. Radiology. 2012 Mar;262(3):781-5.
Israel GM, Bosniak MA. How I do it: evaluating renal masses. Radiology. 2005 Aug;236(2):441-50.

Bosniak Category	Characteristics	Management
I	Water attenuation, nonenhancing	Benign; no follow-up
	No septa, calcifications, or solid components	
II	Few hairline-thin septa in which slight enhancement may be perceptible but not measurable	Essentially always benign; no follow-up
	Fine calcification or short segment of slightly thicker calcification may be present in wall or septa	
	Hyperdense lesions: homogeneous, sharply marginated, nonenhancing, size <3 cm	
IIF	Multiple septa which can be minimally thickened, with slight enhancement that can be perceptible but not measurable	Usually benign; follow-up required to prove stability
	Calcification of the wall or septa may be thick and nodular	
	Hyperdense lesions: homogeneous, sharply marginated, nonenhancing, size >3 cm	
III	Thick and/or irregular wall of lesion with measurable enhancement	Cannot exclude neoplasm; need surgical intervention for histologic diagnosis
IV	Distinct enhancing soft tissue components independent of wall or septa	Definitely malignant; need to be surgically removed

Table I. Bosniak classification system.

Chemical shift and gadolinium-enhanced MRI identifies adrenal adenomas with high specificity and acceptable sensitivity

1. The relative change in mass-liver signal intensity (SI) ratio on opposed-phase versus in-phase magnetic resonance (MR) imaging was highly specific and sensitive in characterizing adrenal masses as adenomas.

2. Adenomas and nonadenomas could not be effectively differentiated with maximum SI after contrast administration or maximum washout.

Original Date of Publication: November 1995

Study Rundown: Adrenal masses are common incidental findings seen on computed tomography and encompass a spectrum of benign and malignant causes. For patients with extra-adrenal primary malignancy, deciphering the nature of concurrent adrenal lesions is critical given that the adrenal glands are in some instances the only site of metastatic disease. In attempting to differentiate adenomas from malignant adrenal masses using MR, the SI ratio of the adrenal mass to liver or fat on T1-weighted (T1W) and T2-weighted (T2W) spin-echo images generated with low- and medium-field strength magnets was initially proposed. However, with significant overlap in ratios for adenomas and nonadenomas, this MR technique proved to be of limited use in identifying malignant adrenal masses. This was until Mitchell and colleagues established that lipid-sensitive chemical shift techniques could be used to identify adrenal adenomas. This was on the basis that benign adrenocortical masses often contain high lipid content, while metastases and pheochromocytomas do not. Adenomas and nonadenomas also have different patterns of gadolinium enhancement.

The present study by Korobkin and colleagues evaluated the use of chemical shift and dynamic gadolinium-enhanced MR imaging in characterizing adrenal masses. Definitive diagnoses were made on the basis of other clinical imaging and pathologic criteria. This study found that a decrease in the relative SI ratio on opposed-phase chemical shift images could be used to identify adenomas with high specificity and acceptable sensitivity. Visual assessment of adrenal masses with maximum SI after gadolinium enhancement did not allow for effective differentiation between adenomas and nonadenomas, and did not improve with washout.

In-Depth [prospective cohort]: Patients with adrenal masses detected through abdominal CT were consecutively enrolled into this study and further evaluated with chemical shift MR imaging, dynamic gadolinium-enhanced MR imaging, or both. Adrenal masses were assessed and defined as either adenomas or nonadenomas on the basis of other non-MR imaging and pathologic criteria. This included NP-59 scintigraphy, which was used to evaluate clinically suspected hyperfunctioning adenomas and some suspected non-hyperfunctioning adenomas. Percutaneous biopsy was performed when the adrenal mass was the only suspected metastatic site from an extra-adrenal primary neoplasm. Quantitative and qualitative review of the MR images was performed, assessing mass-liver SI ratios for T1W and T2W images. The relative change in mass-liver and mass-paraspinal muscle SI ratios on opposed-phase versus in-phase gradient echo (GRE) imaging, the relative change in mass-liver SI ratio on fat-saturated T1W versus conventional T1W imaging, and the maximum SI of adrenal masses on gadolinium-enhanced images were evaluated compared to unenhanced images. Comparing SI at maximum enhancement to that on the final 10 minute image allowed for the assessment of maximum gadolinium washout for each evaluated mass. Qualitative review was conducted using a 5-point scale and carried out by 2 investigators blinded to the clinical history and results of previous non-MR imaging. A single investigator blinded to the clinical data and qualitative results was responsible for quantitative review.

A total of 43 patients with 51 adrenal masses participated in this study. Of the 51 adrenal masses evaluated, 35 (n=28, mean age 57 years, range 35-78 years) were diagnosed as adenomas using non-MR imaging and/or pathology. The remaining 16 masses (n=15, mean age 51 years, range 19-72) were diagnosed as nonadenomas.

Based on the results of qualitative review comparing adenomas and nonadenomas, the relative change in mass-liver ratio SI on opposed-phase versus in-phase GRE images were able to characterize adenomas with 100% specificity and 81% sensitivity. Adenomas were also identified with 100% specificity using the relative change in mass-muscle SI ratio on opposed-phase versus in-phase images (77% sensitivity) and the relative change in mass-liver SI ratio on fat-saturated T1W versus conventional T1W images (30% sensitivity). However, the maximum SI of an adrenal mass after contrast administration and following maximum contrast washout were of little to no diagnostic value, with 100% overlap in SI for adenomas and nonadenomas.

Korobkin M, Lombardi TJ, Aisen AM, Francis IR, Quint LE, Dunnick NR, Londy F, Shapiro B, Gross MD, Thompson NW. Characterization of adrenal masses with chemical shift and gadolinium-enhanced MR imaging. Radiology. 1995 Nov;197(2):411-8.

Additional Review:

Mitchell DG, Crovello M, Matteucci T, Petersen RO, Miettinen MM. Benign adrenocortical masses: diagnosis with chemical shift MR imaging. Radiology. 1992 Nov;185(2):345-51.

Rapid CT contrast washout differentiates adrenal adenomas from nonadenomas

1. The mean percentage of computed tomography (CT) contrast washout was significantly greater for adenomas compared to nonadenomas in all delayed scans.

2. Delayed enhanced CT scans discriminated adenomas from nonadenomas with high sensitivity and specificity at various time points, as early as 5 to 15 minutes after enhancement.

Original Date of Publication: March 1998

Study Rundown: Adrenal mass lesions are incidentally discovered in up to 5% of patients subjected to CT for indications unrelated to adrenal disease. In patients without a known history of cancer, most of these lesions are benign. For patients with a diagnosed extra-adrenal malignancy, the likelihood that an incidentally discovered adrenal lesion is malignant increases considerably. On unenhanced CT scans, benign adrenal adenomas are characterized by low attenuation. On contrast-enhanced CT, however, attenuation values cannot differentiate between benign and malignant lesions. As such, other imaging modalities or repeat imaging have been historically used to differentiate between benign and malignant adrenal masses. This was until several studies noted that intravenous (IV) contrast medium tended to "wash out" faster from adenomatous lesions than non-adenomatous lesions, and therefore, CT attenuation measurements could be used after a variable delay period to characterize adrenal lesions. Given that delayed CT attenuation measurements are dependent on the type, total dose and injection rate of IV contrast material, however, measures of absolute attenuation on delayed scans were found not found to be useful. In response, the use of enhancement washout curves was proposed to differentiate adrenal adenomas from nonadenomas.

In this study conducted by Korobkin and colleagues, contrast enhancement washout curves were generated following delayed contrast-enhanced CT scans of adrenal adenomas and nonadenomas. The results of this study showed that the mean percentage of enhancement washout for adrenal adenomas far exceeded that observed in nonadenomas. The authors also demonstrated that delayed enhanced CT scans could discriminate adenomas from nonadenomas with high sensitivity and specificity at various time points, as early as 5 to 15 minutes after enhancement. Pena and colleagues later confirmed in their study that the relative percentage washout on dynamic and delayed enhanced CT scans could be used to characterize adrenal masses.

In-Depth [prospective cohort]: Patients with adrenal masses identified through abdominal or chest CT were consecutively enrolled into this study. Adrenal adenoma diagnoses were confirmed through various means, including percutaneous biopsy, stable appearance on follow-up CT examinations and an attenuation value of <10 Hounsfield Units (HU) on unenhanced CT. Nonadenoma diagnoses were confirmed through surgery, percutaneous biopsy, substantial growth or shrinkage at short-term follow-up, and stable CT for 1 case of myelolipoma. Unenhanced and standard enhanced scans were obtained for all adrenal masses, and delayed enhanced CT values were studied in 2 groups of patients. In the first group, delayed scans were obtained at 15, 30 and 45 minutes following the initial enhanced CT. In the second group, delayed scans were obtained at 5, 10 and 15 minutes after the initial enhanced CT. From these scans, percentages of initial enhancement at these time points were calculated and used to generate washout curves for adrenal adenomas and nonadenomas. Calculations of sensitivity and specificity for the diagnosis of adenoma using delayed enhanced CT were made after selecting an optimal threshold value.

A total of 66 patients with 76 adrenal masses were evaluated. The masses consisted of 52 adenomas (n=45; mean age 64 years, range 43-80 years; 53% men) and 24 nonadenomas (n=21; mean age 60 years, range 31-76 years; 71% men). Consistent with previous studies, there was no significant difference in mean CT attenuation at initial enhancement for adenomatous versus nonadenomatous masses. However, a statistically significant difference in mean CT attenuation between adenomas and nonadenomas was observed for unenhanced ($p < 0.001$) and all delayed enhanced ($p < 0.001$) scans. For unenhanced scans, an optimal threshold of 10 HU corresponded to a sensitivity of 87% and specificity of 100%. For the 15-minute delayed enhanced scan, the sensitivity and specificity were both 96% at a threshold of 37 HU. Differences in mean percentages of initial enhancement were also found to be statistically significant between the adenoma and nonadenoma groups at all delayed times ($p < 0.001$). The mean percentage of enhancement washout for adrenal adenomas was 51% at 5 minutes and 70% at 15 minutes, compared to 8% and 20% for nonadenomas, respectively. On the 15-minute delayed enhanced scans, an optimal threshold for adenoma diagnosis was established at 60% contrast enhancement washout, associated with a sensitivity of 88% and specificity of 96%.

Korobkin M, Brodeur FJ, Francis IR, Quint LE, Dunnick NR, Londy F. CT time-attenuation washout curves of adrenal adenomas and nonadenomas. American Journal of Roentgenology. 1998 Mar;170(3):747-52.

Additional Review:

Blake MA, Cronin CG, Boland GW. Adrenal imaging. American Journal of Roentgenology. 2010;194(6):1450.

Boland GWL, Blake MA, Hahn PF, Mayo-Smith WW. Incidental Adrenal Lesions: Principles, Techniques, and Algorithms for Imaging Characterization. Radiology. 2008 Dec;249(3):756-75.

Peña CS, Boland GWL, Hahn PF, Lee MJ, Mueller PR. Characterization of Indeterminate (Lipid-poor) Adrenal Masses: Use of Washout Characteristics at Contrast-enhanced CT. Radiology. 2000 Dec;217(3):798-802.

Hepatic arterial phase imaging more sensitive than portal venous phase in the detection of hepatic lesions and arterioportal shunting

1. Hepatic arterial phase imaging detected more hepatic lesions than portal venous phase (PVP) imaging, as well as arterioportal shunting not seen on PVP images.

2. PVP imaging was more sensitive in the detection of portal vein thrombosis due to hepatic tumor invasion.

Original Date of Publication: May 1996

Study Rundown: The administration of contrast has improved the imaging of malignant liver lesions using computed tomography (CT). Some tumors, however, are more difficult to visualize despite the use of contrast, including primary hepatocellular carcinoma (HCC), metastases from renal cell carcinoma, pancreatic islet cell tumors and some cases of breast carcinoma. This can be explained by the increased vascularity of these lesions, which allows for rapid enhancement and subsequent fading to an attenuation similar to background liver parenchyma. In recognizing that the visualization of morphologic CT contrast patterns is largely influenced by techniques of contrast administration, Freeny and colleagues found that benign hepatic hemangiomas could be differentiated from malignant hepatic neoplasms using bolus dynamic scanning. In a later study, Heiken and colleagues established that CT imaging of hepatic tumors could be further improved by performing CT during arterial portography (CTAP) via the superior mesenteric or splenic arteries. This technique allowed for the enhancement of the portal vein and intrahepatic vessels, which proved to be useful in predicting tumor behavior when Matsui and colleagues observed that intranodular portal blood flow decreased with increasing tumor grade. The same study also found that hepatic angiography could be used to identify HCCs as the arterial blood flow to these lesions exceeds that of the surrounding liver. As such, these lesions can be seen early during contrast administration through the aorta or hepatic artery, otherwise known as the hepatic arterial-dominant phase (HAP) of contrast delivery.

In the study conducted by Baron and colleagues, hepatic arterial-dominant phase (HAP) imaging was compared to portal venous-dominant phase (PVP) imaging in the evaluation of HCC. The results of this study showed that considerably more lesions were detected during HAP than PVP, including lesions not seen with PVP imaging. HAP imaging was also able to identify arterioportal shunting, which was not evident in any of the images produced during PVP. Both techniques were able to identify portal venous thrombosis; however, some cases were missed with HAP imaging when compared to PVP imaging. Therefore, the use of both HAP and PVP imaging optimizes the evaluation of patients with or at risk of HCC.

In-Depth [retrospective cohort]: All patients with a proven diagnosis of HCC visualized with biphasic helical CT between 1993 and 1994 were assessed for inclusion in the study (n=78). HCC was confirmed through needle core biopsy, fine-needle aspiration or surgical resection. Patients were excluded if they had received prior iodized oil infusion, or if any technical failures encountered during scanning prohibited the acquisition of PVP images within the required time. Patients eligible for inclusion in the study received either 150 mL of ionic contrast material (iothalamate meglumine 60%) at a rate of 2.5 mL/sec, or nonionic contrast material (ioversol 68%) at a rate of 3-5 mL/sec. As all patients had proven HCC, all lesions with a similar appearance to the lesion sampled for biopsy without meeting CT criteria for hemangiomas, cyst or confluent fibrosis, were also considered tumor nodules. Three investigators retrospectively reviewed all CT scans, and consensus was reached for all cases.

A total of 66 patients (mean age 58 years) were included in this study. Based on the results of both PVP and HAP imaging, 326 lesions were detected with an average of 5 lesions per patient. Of these 326 lesions, PVP images depicted 268 (82%) compared to 309 (95%) on HAP images. For 7 patients, lesions were seen only on HAP images, and not depicted in PVP imaging. However, in 13 patients, PVP images showed additional lesions not seen on HAP imaging. PVP imaging was also more sensitive in the detection of portal venous thrombosis due to tumor invasion, detecting 21 cases compared to 17 on HAP imaging, but not arterioportal shunting. Based on HAP imaging, arterioportal shunting was evident in 11 patients, while no cases were identified through PVP imaging.

Baron RL, J H Oliver r, G D Dodd r, Nalesnik M, Holbert BL, Carr B. Hepatocellular carcinoma: evaluation with biphasic, contrast-enhanced, helical CT. Radiology. 1996 May;199(2):505-11.

Additional Review:

Freeny PC, Marks WM. Patterns of contrast enhancement of benign and malignant hepatic neoplasms during bolus dynamic and delayed CT. Radiology. 1986 Sep;160(3):613-8.

Heiken JP, Weyman PJ, Lee JK, Balfe DM, Picus D, Brunt EM, et al. Detection of focal hepatic masses: prospective evaluation with CT, delayed CT, CT during arterial portography, and MR imaging. Radiology. 1989 Apr;171(1):47-51.

Matsui O, Kadoya M, Kameyama T, Yoshikawa J, Takashima T, Nakanuma Y, Unoura M, Kobayashi K, Izumi R, Ida M. Benign and malignant nodules in cirrhotic livers: distinction based on blood supply. Radiology. 1991 Feb;178(2):493-7.

Magnetic resonance-based preoperative evaluation for perianal fistulas superior to traditional clinical methods, improves surgical outcomes

1. Preoperative magnetic resonance imaging (MRI) requiring no patient preparation has excellent concordance with surgical findings in perianal fistula and aids in surgical planning.

2. MRI is better than initial surgical exploration in the prediction of patient outcomes.

Original Date of Publication: May 2000

Study Rundown: A perianal fistula is an abnormal connection between a primary opening inside the anal canal to a secondary opening in the perianal skin, often from a draining anorectal abscess. The management of perianal fistulas is a challenging issue in colorectal surgery. Surgery is the primary treatment with the aim of draining local infection, removing the fistulous tract, and protecting sphincter function. In addition to preoperative sphincter function, surgical outcome relies on fistula location, type, and duration. Thus, a thorough understanding of anorectal anatomy is imperative before performing surgery.

Perianal fistulas traditionally are classified by location in relation to the external anal sphincter proposed by Park et al. using only the coronal axis (Table I). Clinical examination based on this classification proved superior to many prior tested imaging techniques, including fistulography, anal endosonography, and computed tomography. However, radiologists at the St. James's University Hospital recommended a classification that applies Parks surgical classification to MR imaging findings in both the axial and coronal planes (Table II). This provided a more accurate description of the fistula's relationship to the anatomy of the anal canal and sphincter complex. The St. James's University Hospital classification thus increases the chance of accurate indication for surgery and avoidance of adverse side effects from inaccurate treatment.

In-Depth [classification system based on prospective data]: This prospective study used gradient-echo T1 dynamic gadolinium-enhanced MR imaging to demonstrate and classify perianal fistulas into five grades that were based on Parks's surgical classification. The grades expand on Parks's classification by classifying anatomy based on the axial and coronal planes. Using both planes, MR imaging clearly shows the anatomical location and course of "high" perianal fistulas that are often misdiagnosed by clinical examination. T2-weighted and short-inversion-time inversion recovery (STIR) show pathologic fistulas, secondary fistulous tracks, and fluid collection. STIR imaging occasionally failed to indicate secondary fistulous tracks and small edematous changes.

The St. James's University Hospital classification system was based on 300 patients with surgically proven fistulas. Fistulas were organized into five grades based on increasing severity: grade 1, simple linear intersphincteric fistula; grade 2, intersphincteric fistula with abscess or secondary tract; grade 3, trans-sphincteric fistula; grade 4, trans-sphincteric fistula with abscess or secondary tract within the ischiorectal fossa; grade 5, supralevator and translevator disease. Patient outcome was predicated on whether further surgery was indicated after MR imaging. Use of this classification indicated a significant correlation with patient outcome ($p < 0.001$). MR imaging grades 1 and 2 were associated with no indication for surgery and MR imaging grades 3-5 were associated with indication for surgery. The study concluded that any tract or abscess in the ischiorectal fossa is related to a complex fistula indicating the need for surgery (grades 3-5).

Morris J, Spencer JA, Ambrose NS. MR Imaging Classification of Perianal Fistulas and Its Implications for Patient Management. RadioGraphics. 2000 May 1;20(3):623–35.

Parks AG, Gordon PH, Hardcastle JD. A classification of fistula-in-ano. Br J Surg. 1976 Jan 1;63(1):1–12.

Type	Description and subtypes
I	Intersphincteric - Simple low track - High track - High track with rectal opening - Extra rectal extension
II	Trans-sphincteric - Uncomplicated - High track
III	Suprasphincteric - Uncomplicated - High track
IV	Extrasphincteric - Secondary to trauma - Secondary to anorectal disease - Secondary to pelvic inflammation

Table I. Parks Classification. Underneath each major classification are subtypes. Unlike the St. James classification, complications are associated with each type.

Grade	Description
1	Simple linear intersphincteric fistula
2	Intersphincteric fistula with abscess or secondary track
3	Trans-sphincteric fistula
4	Trans-sphincteric fistula with abscess or secondary track within the ischiorectal fossa
5	Supralevator and translevator disease

Table II. St. James's Classification. Grades 1 and 2 were strongly correlated with no subsequent surgery, while grades 3-5 strongly correlated with surgical intervention.

MRI offers an alternative to endoscopic assessment of disease activity and severity in ileocolonic Crohn's disease

1. Magnetic resonance imaging (MRI) offers an effective alternative to endoscopy for quantifying disease severity in Crohn's disease.

2. MRI required 3T field strength, both oral and rectal contrast, IV antiperistalsis medication, and IV contrast administration.

Original Date of Publication: January 2009

Study Rundown: Appropriate therapy of Crohn's disease depends on disease severity and complications. The variable lifelong clinical course therefore necessitates frequent and accurate evaluation of disease activity. Historically, the diagnostic gold standard for Crohn's disease is based on endoscopic findings coupled with biochemical markers (such as faecal calprotectin (fC) and C-reactive protein (CRP)) and clinical scores (Harvey-Bradshaw Index (HBI) and Crohn's disease activity index (CDAI)). Endoscopy, however, can only access the proximal small bowel or terminal ileum. Imaging modalities have consequently been evaluated. Computed tomography (CT) enterography is accurate but results in ionizing radiation exposure. Transabdominal ultrasound lacks sensitivity and specificity, has high interobserver variability, and is limited by overlying bowel gas. Magnetic resonance (MR) imaging, due to its lack ionizing radiation exposure and high sensitivity and specificity, is being increasingly utilized in the diagnosis of Crohn's disease.

There was previously a lack of definitive criteria to evaluate Crohn's disease based on MR parameters. In a 2008 cross-sectional study done at the Hospital Clinic de Barcelona, a Magnetic Resonance Index of Activity (MaRIA) using wall signal intensity (WSI), relative contrast enhancement (RCE), edema, and presence of ulcers was internally validated as an independent predictor of Crohn's disease severity. The same researchers externally validated the MaRIA 3 years layer. Given the segmental predictors the MaRIA uses, however, it may fail to appreciate the wide-ranging complications and total disease burden of Crohn's disease. In a 2013 prospective trial by Makanyanga et al., a magnetic resonance enterography global score (MEGS) was internally validated against fC and CRP. Used in conjunction, the measures provide an accurate assessment of the activity and severity of Crohn's disease.

In-Depth [cross-sectional]: This study assessed 50 patients with clinically active (n=35) or inactive (n=15) Crohn's disease based on the HBI. Ileocolonoscopy was used as the reference standard against MR. Except for a small number of patients, both assessments were performed the same day. Ileoendoscopic lesions were classified according to Crohn's Disease Endoscopic Index of Severity (CDEIS). MR imaging was performed using a 3.0 T unit after bowel preparation and after oral ingestion of a large volume of polyethylene glycol. Additionally, saline was administered rectally and IV anti peristaltic medication was given. IV gadolinium was also administered. Bowel wall thickness, ulceration, edema, pseudopolyp identification, lymph node enlargement, WSI before and after contrast, and RCE were analyzed. The chi-square test, ANOVA followed by the Bonferoni posthoc test, and Spearman rank coefficient were used for statistical analysis; results were subsequently internally validated using bootstrap bagging with 1000 samples. All paired MR evaluations were performed by two radiologists for interobserver agreement.

Complete endoscopic evaluation was completed in 36 patients (72% of total), yielding 213 colonic segments. MR and endoscopic findings were highly correlated for all parameters and interobserver agreement was very high ($p < 0.001$ for all). Wall thickness ($p < 0.001$), RCE ($p = 0.013$), and ulcer identification ($p = 0.003$) at MR were found to be independent predictors of active disease based on logistic regression analysis, with a sensitivity of 0.9 and specificity of 0.94. The MaRIA index was calculated to have a high ($r = 0.81$) and significant ($p < 0.001$) correlation with the CDEIS of each analogous colonic segment. Overall, the index has a high accuracy for detecting Crohn's disease activity (sensitivity 0.81, specificity 0.89) and for detecting ulcerative lesions (sensitivity 0.95, specificity 0.91) in the colon and terminal ileum.

Rimola J, Rodriguez S, García-Bosch O, Ordás I, Ayala E, Aceituno M, et al. Magnetic resonance for assessment of disease activity and severity in ileocolonic Crohn's disease. Gut. 2009 Aug 1;58(8):1113–20.

Additional Review:

Makanyanga JC, Pendsé D, Dikaios N, Bloom S, McCartney S, Helbren E, et al. Evaluation of Crohn's disease activity: Initial validation of a magnetic resonance enterography global score (MEGS) against faecal calprotectin. Eur Radiol. 2014 Feb 1;24(2):277–87.

Rimola J, Ordás I, Rodriguez S, García-Bosch O, Aceituno M, Llach J, et al. Magnetic resonance imaging for evaluation of Crohn's disease: validation of parameters of severity and quantitative index of activity. Inflamm Bowel Dis. 2011 Aug;17(8):1759–68.

Variable	Scoring
Deep ulceration	0 if absent, 12 if present
Superficial ulceration	0 if absent, 6 if present
Length of ulcerated mucosa	0-10, according to length in centimeters
Length of diseased mucosa	0-10, according to length in centimeters
Stenosis present	3 points if ulcerated stenosis; further 3 points if nonulcerated

Table I. Crohn's Disease Endoscopic Index of Severity (CDEIS): The first four endoscopic variables are scored for the following locations: rectum; sigmoid and left colon; transverse colon; right colon; and ileum. Total score is divided by number of locations.

Variable	Description
Bowel wall thickness	Measured in mm
Mucosal ulceration	Presence of deep depressions in mucosal surface
Mural edema	Presence of hyperintensity on T2-wedged sequences of the colon wall relative to the signal of the psoas muscle
Pseudopolyps in the lumen	Presence or absence
Enlarged regional lymph nodes	Greater than 1 cm
Wall signal intensity (WSI)	Quantitative measurement before and after IV contrast administration
Relative contrast enhancement (RCE)	RCE = (WSI postgadolinium – WSI pregadolinium) x 100 x (SD noise pregadolinium/SD noise postgadolinium)

Table II: Magnetic Resonance Index of Activity: Variables used in the statistical validation of the MaRIA index. Note that SD noise corresponds to the average of three SDs of the signal intensity measured outside the body before and after gadolinium injection. The same segmentation is used as in the CDEIS.

	0	1	2	3
Mural thickness	<3 mm	3-5 mm	5-7 mm	>7 mm
Mural T2 signal	Equal to normal bowel wall	Minor increase in signal	Moderate increase in signal	Marked increase in signal
Per-mural T2 signal	Equal to normal mesentery	Increase in mesenteric signal but no fluid	Small fluid rim	Large fluid rim (>2 mm)
T1 enhancement	Equal to normal bowel	Minor enhancement	Moderate enhancement	Marked enhancement
Mural enhancement pattern	N/A or homogenous	Mucosal	Layered	
Haustral loss (colon only)	None	<1/3 segment	1/3-2/3 segment	>2/3 segment
Multiplication factor per segment based on length of segment		0-5 cm x 1	5-15 cm x 1.5	>15 cm x 2
	Additional extramural features that, when present, increase score by 5 points: lymph nodes, Comb sign, abscess, fistulae			

Table III. Magnetic Resonance Enterography Global Score (MEGS): A total score is calculated based the points (top row) for each given variable (left column). The same segments are evaluated as in the MaRIA index and CDEIS.

Visualization of noncystic masses on transvaginal ultrasound sensitive and specific for ectopic pregnancy

1. Sonographic demonstration of any non-cystic adnexal mass is both sensitive and specific for in the diagnosis of ectopic pregnancy (EP) by transvaginal ultrasonography (TVUS).

2. Visualization of a non-cystic adnexal mass is comparably specific to direct imaging of a living extrauterine pregnancy or gestational sac, but significantly more sensitive for EP.

Original Date of Publication: April 1994

Study Rundown: EP is life threatening obstetric emergency in which gestation occurs outside the uterus, often presenting as an acute onset of pelvic pain with vaginal bleeding. The majority of EPs occur within the fallopian tube, but the embryo may also implant within the cervix, ovaries, or abdomen, and may require emergent laparoscopic removal in any of these locations. Accurate diagnosis includes both the measurement of serum human chorionic gonadotropin levels to confirm pregnancy and ultrasonographic visualization of ectopic products of conception, as confirmed by the works of Shalev et al., Condous et al., and Gracia and Barnhart. Once multiple studies confirmed the appropriateness of TVUS as the first-line study in the diagnosis of EP, the question arose regarding what must specifically be visualized at the threshold of positivity to most sensitively and specifically diagnose EP. The referenced study reviewed and meta-analyzed the contemporary literature to determine which of four criteria, in descending order of stringency, was most appropriate to use as the broad threshold for TVUS positivity in the diagnosis of EP. The four criteria reviewed were, at the most stringent, (1) direct visualization of a living extrauterine pregnancy, followed by (2) an extrauterine gestational sac with yolk sac or embryo, (3) an empty tubal ring, or extrauterine fluid collection with a surrounding hyperechoic ring, or (4) any adnexal mass other than a simple cyst, allowing inclusion of visualized hematoma in addition to any products of conception. The authors found that while the more stringent criteria were most specific (99-100%), they were highly insensitive (20-65%), and bore only moderate negative predictive values (NPVs, 78-89%). The least stringent criterion traded a minimally decreased specificity (98.9%) for a significant improvement in sensitivity (84%) and NPV (95%). By these criteria, TVUS interpretation in the diagnosis of EP was simplified, thereby reducing failures to diagnose a potentially fatal condition while improving early recognition of EP and increasing opportunities for medical management with methotrexate over laparoscopic intervention. Notably, this study did not evaluate the effect on visualization of free fluid within the peritoneum, which may occur following rupture of an EP, but nonetheless established the most sensitive and specific criterion by which to interpret TVUS in the diagnosis of EP.

In-Depth [systematic review and meta-analysis]: This systematic review and meta-analysis pooled data from studies published between 1986 and 1993 examining the use of TVUS in the diagnostic workup of patients with suspected EP. A total of 2216 patients (1651 with EP, and 565 without) spanning 10 studies were included in which all enrolled patients were assessed by TVUS in the workup for EP with subsequent surgical confirmation of all cases. Sensitivity, specificity, positive predictive values (PPVs) and NPVs were calculated using Bayes' theorem for each of four different positivity criteria used as the diagnostic threshold in TVUS assessment. Given that EPs may be visualized as anything ranging from an intact extrauterine pregnancy to an adnexal hematoma or other complex adnexal mass, the four tested criteria sought to encompass a stepwise progression in sonographic specificity as follows: the most stringent criterion required visualization of an extrauterine embryo with a heartbeat (20.1% sensitivity, 100% specificity, NPV 78.5%); followed by an extrauterine gestational sac with yolk sac or embryo (36.6% sensitivity, 100% specificity, NPV 82.2%); an adnexal mass with a central anechoic region or hyperechoic rim, known as an "empty tubal ring" (64.6% sensitivity, 99.5% specificity, NPV 89.1%); or the least stringent criterion, any adnexal mass other than a simple cyst or intraovarian lesion (84.4% sensitivity, 98.9% specificity, NPV 94.8%). As the threshold for positivity became less stringent, the sensitivity dramatically increased, yet with minimal decrease in overall specificity, finding that TVUS performed best using the least stringent threshold when EP is suspected. This study established the simplest and most effective interpretation strategy for TVUS in the diagnosis of EP for both presurgical and medical management, and created an interpretative baseline for comparison to alternative diagnostic techniques.

Brown DL, Doubilet PM. Transvaginal sonography for diagnosing ectopic pregnancy: positivity criteria and performance characteristics. JUM. 1994 Apr 1;13(4):259–66.

Additional Review:

Shalev, E, Yarom I, Bustan M, Weiner E, Ben-Shlomo I. Transvaginal sonography as the ultimate diagnostic tool for the management of ectopic pregnancy: experience with 840 cases. Fertility and Sterility. 1998 Jan 1;69(1)62–5.

Condous G, Okaro E, Khalid A, Lu C, Van Huffel S, Timmerman D, Bourne T. The accuracy of transvaginal ultrasonography for the diagnosis of ectopic pregnancy prior to surgery. Human Reproduction. 2005 Feb 3;20(5):1404-09.

Gracia CR, Barnhart KT. Diagnosing ectopic pregnancy: decision analysis comparing six strategies. Obstetrics & Gynecology. 2001 Mar 1;97(3)464-70.

Ultrasonographic compressibility sensitive and specific for deep venous thrombosis

1. Compared to contrast venography, real-time B-mode ultrasound was highly sensitive and specific for the diagnosis of deep venous thrombosis (DVT) based on the single criterion of venous compressibility by the transducer probe.

2. Sensitivity for thrombosis was highest in proximal deep veins of the lower extremity (i.e., the femoral and popliteal veins) and was decreased in detection of thrombosis in isolated distal calf veins.

Original Date of Publication: February 1989

Study Rundown: DVT is a common diagnosis among hospitalized patients due to immobility, hypercoagulable states, and vascular endothelial disruption. Clinical signs and symptoms such as unilateral limb edema, superficial varicosities or tenderness along the deep venous system often prompt consideration of a diagnosis of DVT, but physical examination remains a highly unreliable diagnostic technique even in the setting of significant risk factors. Given the high risk of anticoagulation as a treatment for DVT, confirmatory imaging remains a necessity even in light of modern risk stratification systems such as the Well's criteria. The gold-standard imaging modality for DVT is contrast venography, an invasive procedure in which a contrast agent is directly introduced to the venous system and viewed under fluoroscopy for a luminal filling defect. Several less invasive methods were tested as diagnostic alternatives, including impedance plethysmography and Doppler ultrasonography, but with the referenced article, these techniques were supplanted by B-mode ultrasound, which allowed direct, non-invasive visualization of the deep venous system.

This study was the first to prospectively compare the results of B-mode ultrasonographic examination to those of contrast venography in patients with suspected DVT. The authors utilized the single criterion of absent venous compressibility for determination of positivity on an ultrasound examination, finding it to be both highly sensitive and specific within the proximal deep venous system as compared to contrast venography. However, sensitivity was limited in the more distal calf veins, particularly when these vessels were thrombosed in isolation. Notably, this study was performed in a sampling of outpatients, though the results were subsequently confirmed among hospitalized patients, making bedside B-mode ultrasound the first line tool to either rule-in or rule-out DVT in any care setting.

In-Depth [prospective cohort]: This prospective trial enrolled 220 consecutive outpatients (median age 56 years; 56% female) in Italy and Holland for routine contrast venography after clinical concern for lower extremity DVT was raised during outpatient examination. Exclusion criteria included anticoagulation within 48 hours, contrast allergy, or prior diagnosis of DVT within 1 year of examination. Each patient underwent B-mode ultrasonography of the common femoral and popliteal veins, followed by contrast venography within 2 hours performed by a radiologist blinded to the results of the ultrasound examination. Venous compressibility on ultrasound examination was determined by simple application of pressure by the transducer probe, with a lack of visible venous compression being considered visual evidence of thrombus. The presence of intraluminal echogenic bands within the vessel and changes in venous diameter during performance of a Valsalva maneuver by the patient were also assessed as potential criteria for DVT during ultrasonography. All ultrasound results were reviewed by two independent radiologists, and were found to be in complete agreement ($\kappa = 1$). Additionally, ultrasonographic exams of 45 patients were repeated by a separate examiner blinded to the results of the initial examination, revealing complete interobserver agreement for venous compressibility ($\kappa = 1$).

B-mode ultrasound using venous compressibility as the sole criterion for the presence of proximal DVT was 100% sensitive (95%CI 95-100%; n=66). When including patients with additional calf-vein thromboses, the overall sensitivity fell to 91%. In cases of isolated distal calf vein thrombosis, the sensitivity fell to 36% (n=11). All patients without DVT on venography had fully compressible common femoral veins (n=143), with only a single patient showing non-compressibility of the popliteal vein (n=142), resulting in a specificity of 99% (95%CI 97-100%). Other possible criteria of positivity on ultrasonography, such as the presence of intraluminal echogenic bands or change in venous diameter during Valsalva were found to be of low specificity for DVT (52% and 67%, respectively), though the former was highly sensitive (99%). Taken together, this study revealed, with a high degree of interobserver reliability, that venous compressibility visualized by B-mode ultrasound was 91% sensitive and 99% specific for the presence of DVT among outpatients.

Lensing AW, Prandoni P, Brandjes D, Huisman PM, Vigo M, Tomasella G, et al. Detection of Deep-Vein Thrombosis by Real-Time B-Mode Ultrasonography. The New England Journal of Medicine. 1989 Feb 9;320(6):342–45.

Compression ultrasound identifies proximal deep venous thrombosis with high sensitivity and specificity

1. Vein compressibility assessed with ultrasonography (US) was highly sensitive and specific for the diagnosis of proximal-vein deep vein thrombosis (DVT) when compared to contrast venography.

2. Isolated calf-vein thrombosis could not be reliably detected through compression US.

Original Date of Publication: February 1989

Study Rundown: DVT refers to the formation of a blood clot within a deep vein, most commonly at or above the knee, such as the popliteal, femoral and iliac veins. If left untreated, patients are at risk for fatal pulmonary embolism. Diagnosis based on clinical signs and symptoms, however, is unreliable, necessitating the use of more objective testing. Historically, this has included contrast material phlebography, a technique that was later replaced by non-invasive tests such as phleborheography and impedance plethysmography. Impedance plethysmography reliably identifies occlusive thrombi in the proximal veins (popliteal, femoral or iliac veins), but is less reliable in the detection of non-occlusive proximal DVT and thrombi found in the calf. As such, other methods of DVT detection emerged, including US. While many different US diagnostic criteria had been initially proposed, Cronon and colleagues demonstrated that vein compressibility assessed through US could be used with high sensitivity and specificity in detecting DVT.

In this larger prospective study later conducted by Lensing and colleagues, gold standard contrast venography was compared to real-time B-mode US using the single criterion of vein compressibility. The results of this study showed that US had high sensitivity and specificity in the detection of proximal-vein thrombosis. Isolated calf-vein thrombosis, however, was not reliably detected through US, limiting its sensitivity for thrombi in this location. The study also found visualization of an echogenic band in the proximal veins to be a highly sensitive but non-specific criterion for proximal-vein thrombosis. Changes in vein diameter during the Valsalva maneuver were neither sensitive nor specific.

In-Depth [prospective cohort]: All outpatients with suspected DVT were referred for evaluation and consecutively screened for enrollment (n=233). Key exclusion criteria included anticoagulant treatment for more than 48 hours before referral, known allergy to contrast material, or a recent episode of DVT in the past year. Following screening and consent, each patient underwent US of the symptomatic leg, where only the common femoral and popliteal veins were scanned. Compressibility of both veins was considered a negative test result, while non-compressibility of one or more veins was considered positive for venous thrombosis. Contrast venography was subsequently performed within 2 hours of US and interpreted by a radiologist blinded to the results of US. In a subset of 45 patients, US was repeated by an independent examiner to determine interobserver agreement on compressibility.

Contrast venography and US was successfully performed in a total of 220 patients (median age 56 years, range 17-86; 56% women). Based on the reference standard (venography), 66 patients were found to have proximal-vein thrombosis. Calf-vein thrombosis was confirmed in 11 patients. On US, all 66 cases with proximal-vein thrombosis were found to have non-compressible common femoral veins, popliteal veins or both. Therefore, the sensitivity of US in detecting proximal-vein thrombosis through non-compressibility was 100% (95%CI 95-100%). Of the 143 patients without DVT on venography, 142 had fully compressible proximal veins on US, yielding a specificity of 99% (95%CI 97-100%). The sensitivity of US in detecting calf-vein thrombosis, however, was limited to only 36% (95%CI 11-70%). Interobserver agreement on compressibility was 100% (kappa = 1). The study also found visualization of an echogenic band in the proximal veins to be highly sensitive (99%) but not specific (52%) in DVT detection. The percent change in vein diameter during Valsalva maneuver proved to be of limited use in detecting DVT with a sensitivity and specificity of 55% and 67%, respectively.

Lensing AW, Prandoni P, Brandjes D, Huisman PM, Vigo M, Tomasella G, et al. Detection of deep-vein thrombosis by real-time B-mode ultrasonography. The New England Journal of Medicine. 1989 Feb;320(6):342-5.

Additional Review:

Cronan JJ, Dorfman GS, Scola FH, Schepps B, Alexander J. Deep venous thrombosis: US assessment using vein compression. Radiology. 1987 Jan;162(1):191-4.

Fewer adverse drug reactions occur with nonionic than ionic contrast media

1. The prevalence of adverse drug reactions (ADRs) with the use of intravenous high-osmolar, ionic contrast media was over four-fold greater compared to low-osmolar, nonionic contrast.

2. Severe reactions, including dyspnea, hypotension, cardiac arrest and syncope occurred in over five times as many patients administered ionic media as compared to those administered nonionic media.

Original Date of Publication: June 1990

Study Rundown: Contrast agents, like any intravenously administered drug, pose a significant risk of immediate ADRs ranging from mild nausea, vomiting, pruritus or urticaria to severe and life-threatening reactions such as anaphylaxis or cardiac arrest. Prior to the widespread introduction of nonionic contrast agents in the 1980s, ionic agents were the only available contrast media for contrast-enhanced examinations or angiography, and the value of transitioning to the newer, unqualified agents was questioned on the basis of cost versus a potentially marginal safety benefit. The present study sought to determine if the use of nonionic over ionic agents would improve the safety of contrast-enhanced examinations through a large-scale prospective cohort during a transition period in Japan in which both agents would be in active use.

Including 330 000 cases over three years, the prevalence of any ADRs with the use of intravenous high-osmolar, ionic contrast media was 12.66% as opposed to 3.13% for low-osmolar, nonionic contrast media. Severe ADRs requiring immediate treatment occurred in 0.22% of patients administered ionic contrast media versus 0.04% of those administered nonionic agents. The most significant risk factors for the occurrence of ADRs included young age (less than 30), a history of atopy or other allergy, and a history of cardiac disease. These findings corroborated, on a large-scale, prior findings that the use of nonionic over ionic contrast agents posed a significant improvement in patient safety with regard to the occurrence of all ADRs, and even more importantly, the occurrence of severe and life-threatening ADRs at any level of baseline patient risk. Notably, this study did not examine the risk of contrast-induced nephropathy with these agents, instead focusing primarily on anaphylactic and anaphylactoid reactions.

In-Depth [prospective cohort]: This trial was conducted at 198 institutions across Japan over a period of three years and included 337 647 cases, during which both ionic (50.1% of cases) and nonionic (49.9% of cases) contrast agents were available and in current use in the country. The study was restricted to examinations utilizing intravenous contrast administration only. Cases were excluded if patients underwent examinations other than contrast-enhanced CT, intravenous urography or intravenous digital subtraction angiography, or if records of the ADR or contrast medium were incomplete. ADRs were recorded using a standardized event reporting form by the examining physician at each institution, and were reported at an average rate of 67.8% (range 59.1%-82.3%) independent of patient criteria. ADRs were defined as the acute onset of nausea, vomiting, sensation of heat, urticaria, flushing, vascular pain, hoarseness, coughing, sneezing, chest or abdominal pain, palpitations, rigors, or facial edema. Severe ADRs were defined by dyspnea, sudden hypotension, cardiac arrest or loss of consciousness.

The overall prevalence of all ADRs was significantly lower for ionic (12.66%) versus nonionic (3.13%) contrast agents ($p < 0.01$). An even greater difference was appreciated for severe reactions, at 0.22% for ionic (n=367) versus 0.04% (n=70) for nonionic media ($p < 0.01$). A single fatality occurred in each group, but they were not clearly causally associated with contrast administration. Over 70% of ADRs occurred within 5 minutes of contrast administration in either group. Subgroup analysis revealed that no significant differences in the prevalence of ADRs occurred according to sex or mode of injection. Groups with the greatest prevalence of severe ADRs included those with a history of prior reaction to contrast media (0.73% for ionic versus 0.18% for nonionic agents), a history of general allergy (0.53% for ionic versus 0.10% for nonionic agents) or atopy (0.49% for ionic versus 0.11% for nonionic agents), a history of cardiac disease (0.53% for ionic versus 0.10% for nonionic agents), and those aged 20-29 (0.24% for ionic versus 0.06% for nonionic agents.) Premedication with steroids, antihistamines or sedatives had a positive effect only on the prevalence of severe reactions for ionic agents, but not for nonionic agents. Lastly, subgroups receiving more than 80 mL of ionic contrast showed the lowest prevalence of ADRs (9.9-11.32%), while among those receiving nonionic contrast, the prevalence of ADRs was lowest for the subgroup receiving 81-100 mL (2.50%).

Katayama H, Yamaguchi K, Kozuka T, Takashima T, Seez P, Matsuura K. Adverse Reactions to Ionic and Nonionic Contrast Media, A Report from the Japanese Committee on the Safety of Contrast Media. Radiology. 1990 Jun 175:621–28.

Gadolinium-containing contrast associated with nephrogenic fibrosing dermopathy and systemic fibrosis

1. Among patients with end-stage renal disease (ESRD), gadolinium (Gd) containing magnetic resonance imaging (MRI) contrast agents were found to trigger nephrogenic fibrosing dermopathy (NFD) or nephrogenic systemic fibrosis (NSF) within 1 month of administration.

2. The half-life of gadolinium is dramatically prolonged in ESRD and, when combined with metabolic acidosis, may contribute to dissociation of the Gd-ligand complex and allow tissue precipitation of Gd salts.

Original Date of Publication: June 2006

Study Rundown: Gadolinium-containing contrast agents are used in MRI examinations to reduce the T1 relaxation time of water molecules as they intermittently bind to the paramagnetic metal center, providing increased MR signal. They are typically considered very safe agents even among those with renal insufficiency, with a low rate of adverse reactions and a half-life of roughly 2 hours in those without kidney disease. However, among patients with impaired renal function, that half-life may extend to as long as 120 hours, and it has been proposed that this prolonged exposure may lead to Gd-salt deposition within body tissues and subsequent complications, such as NFD or NSF. NFD is an acquired, idiopathic disease of those with renal failure characterized by painful thickening and induration of the skin, particularly in the distal extremities. NSF is a variant of the same disease in which there is systemic involvement beyond the skin, affecting the joints, lungs, heart or liver.

The present study described a case-control series in which patients with ESRD underwent Gd-enhanced MR angiography (MRA) and developed symptoms of either NFD or NSF, and was among the first publications to describe the association between Gd and these diseases. Of the 9 patients who underwent Gd-enhanced MRA over 2 years, 5 developed skin symptoms suggestive of NFD with characteristic histopathological changes. The most significant differences between those who developed symptoms and those who did not were the presence of a significant metabolic acidosis and a prolonged history of dialysis among those affected versus those unaffected. Despite the inherent limitations of a case-control series study examining a rare disease entity with limited sampling, this study introduced a now common association between Gd-contrast agents and NFD or NSF among ESRD patients.

In-Depth [case-control study]: This series identified 9 dialysis-dependent patients (mean age 58±10.3 years) over a 2-year period who underwent Gd-enhanced MRA with gadopentetic acid, 5 of whom developed skin symptoms suggestive of NFD with characteristic histopathological changes. Baseline characteristics of those affected were compared to those unaffected in an effort to identify potential risk factors for the development of NFD or NSF. In each index case, skin changes occurred 2-4 weeks following the initial administration of gadopentetic acid, and clinical courses were uneventful. Only two major differences were identified between the two patient groups: their mean time on dialysis and their pH values. Those affected had a mean time on dialysis of 36±16.5 months versus 23.75±12.5 months for those unaffected. Additionally, those affected uniformly displayed a metabolic acidosis with an average pH of 7.29±0.04 and serum bicarbonate of 19.5±1.7 mmol/L versus 7.39±0.01 and 22.95±0.58 mmol/L respectively, for those unaffected. A laboratory review including antinuclear antibodies, antineutrophil cytoplasmic antibodies, antiphospholipid antibodies, immune complexes, anti-glomerular basement membrane antibodies and complement factors were unremarkable among both those affected and unaffected. A single affected patient displayed decreased levels of protein C and increased levels of Factor VIII. No medications were identified in common between any of the nine patients.

In those with ESRD, the half-life of Gd-containing compounds is significantly prolonged, and multiple metabolic derangements are often present including metabolic acidosis. This may predispose to dissociation of the Gd ion from its contrast complex, allowing formation of Gd-salts with free anions such as phosphate, which is often increased in concentration in dialysis patients. It was proposed, though without direct evidence, that these salts may precipitate into tissues and trigger the symptoms of NFD or NSF in susceptible patients.

Grobner T. Gadolinium – a specific trigger for the development of nephrogenic fibrosing dermopathy and nephrogenic systemic fibrosis? Nephrology Dialysis Transplantation. 2006 Jan 21:1104–08.

CT utilization associated with future cancer risk

1. Risk projection models estimated 29 000 potential excess cancers related to computed tomography (CT) scans performed in the United States in 2007.

2. Efforts to reduce overall radiation dose from CT, including reduction of unnecessary scans and reducing dose per procedure, continue to be a high priority.

Original Date of Publication: December 2009

Study Rundown: CT has revolutionized medical practice through its speed, availability, and high resolution of anatomical structures free of superimposition. Given its advantages and relative safety over exploratory surgery, its use as a preventative and diagnostic tool for cancer has increased dramatically in the United States since its introduction in the 1970s. However, the nature of CT exposes patients to larger radiation doses than conventional x-ray imaging. As a result, the average radiation dose per United States resident per year has correspondingly increased. The benefits of CT are clear and the radiobiological harm of a single scan are likely insignificant. However, a 2009 retrospective cross-sectional study by Smith-Bindman et al. found that radiation doses from CT scans are higher and more variable than reported. The risk of cumulative CT scans in the patient population may be overlooked and be a cause for public health concern.

While evaluation of the increased risk for cancer from CT is controversial, studies have revived concerns about the risk it poses for developing cancer. In the present cross-sectional study conducted by de González et al., risk models based on cancer rates among survivors of the atomic bomb blasts of World War II (WWII) were used to show a significant number of cancers were likely related to the radiation from CT scans. Using both CT scan frequency and organ-specific doses, the study further indicated that cancers associated with the most frequently used CT scans (abdomen and pelvis) and highest-dose scans (chest CT angiography) had the strongest correlation with cancer risk. Though potentially misleading due to the data set used, the results indicate a substantial possible increased risk of cancer.

In-Depth [cross-sectional]: This epidemiologic study primarily used Medicare claims data, the IMV Medical Information survey of CT scan use in 2007, and a national commercial insurance database (NCID) to estimate the age and gender distribution for CT scan frequency in the United States. Linear extrapolation was used to exclude the estimated scans on those who did not survive 5 years and those with an associated diagnosis code of cancer. Organ-specific doses were based on the Food and Drug Administration's National Evaluation of X-Ray Trends survey and cross checked with an available literature review. Pediatric scans were assumed to follow the recommended lower radiation protocols. Risk models (excluding breast and thyroid) were based on cancer rates among the long-term survivors of the Japanese atomic bomb of WWII. Risk calculations were run using Monte Carlo simulation methods. A no threshold linear model was used.

After excluding scans on patients not surviving greater than 5 years and patients with a cancer diagnosis (gross total of 72 million), an estimated 57 million CT scans were used in the calculation for future cancer risk. Overall, an estimated 29 000 (95%UL 15 000 – 45 000) future cancers were linked to CT scans in the United States in 2007. Abdomen and pelvis (n=14 000, 95%UL 6900 – 25 000), chest (n=4100, 95%UL 1900-8100), and head (n=4000, 95%UL 1100-8700) were found to be scan types performed most frequently. Chest CT angiography (n=2700, 95%UL 1300-5000) was found to be the highest-dose scan. Women were found to have increased radiation exposure due to higher frequency of use (60%) and higher incidence of breast and lung cancer, which require higher-dose scans. The risk models showed lung cancer as the most common radiation associated cancer (n=6200, 95%UL 2300-13 000), primarily due to the high frequency of exposure from chest CT. This was followed by colon cancer (n=3500, 95%UL 1000-6800) due to the high frequency of abdominal CT, and leukemia (n=2800, 95%UL 800-4800) due to high organ sensitivity. Multiple measures to reduce overall population dose, including more widespread use of American College of Radiology (ACR) appropriateness criteria, dose reduction software in CT, Image Gently and Image Wisely, and the development of dose registries have all been instituted.

de González AB, Mahesh M, Kim KP, Bhargavan M, Lewis R, Mettler F, Land C. Projected cancer risks from computed tomographic scans performed in the United States in 2007. Archives of Internal Medicine. 2009 Dec;169(22):2071-2077.

Additional Review:

Smith-Bindman R, Lipson J, Marcus R, Kim KP, Mahesh M, Gould R, et al. Radiation dose associated with common computed tomography examinations and the associated lifetime attributable risk of cancer. Archives of internal medicine. 2009 Dec 14;169(22):2078-2086.

CT scans increase the risk of malignancy in children and young adults

1. In this retrospective cohort analysis of children and young adults without previous malignancy, patients exposed to multiple computed tomography (CT) scans had over 3 times the risk of developing leukemia and brain tumors.

Original Date of Publication: August 2012

Study Rundown: While the connection between radiation exposure and malignancy was previously identified, research on the subject matter drew from high-dose radiation exposure secondary to atomic bombs in Japan. At the time of its publication, this study was the first to use a cohort to examine the malignancy risk associated with low-dose radiation from CT scans. Through retrospective analysis, researchers investigated the relationship between CT-induced radiation exposure during childhood and young adulthood and development of leukemia and brain cancer, as these malignancies occur in particularly radiosensitive tissue. Children under the age of 15 who received 5-10 head CTs were exposed to around 50 milligrays (mGy) of radiation to their marrow, while 2-3 head CTs exposed these children to about 60 mGy of brain radiation. For comparison, the average chest radiograph exposes a child to 0.05 to 0.3 mGy.

Investigators reported an over 3 times increased risk of developing leukemia with exposure to ≥30 mGy and developing a brain tumor with ≥50 mGy of radiation. Limitations included using standardized CT machine settings as a proxy when assessing radiation exposure due to missing data regarding machine-specific settings. However, the use of a cohort from Great Britain's national database ensured a large study group with low risk of loss to follow-up. This was the first cohort study to investigate the potential association between lower doses of radiation than the estimated 100 mGy of radiation exposure experienced by many Japanese atomic bomb victims. While the overall incidence of these malignancies is small within the pediatric population, this study does indicate significant risks associated with over-imaging developing children. With this in mind, the Alliance for Radiation Safety in Pediatric Imaging within the United States has started the "Image Gently" campaign, a movement designed to increase awareness of healthcare practitioners and caregivers to the benefits of reducing unnecessary radiation exposure.

In-Depth [retrospective cohort]: A total of 355 191 patients seen at a Great Britain National Health Service hospital without a history of prior malignancy, but who underwent a first CT scan between 1985-2002 at ages younger than 22, were included in the study. The study group was divided such that 178 604 patients were investigated with respect to leukemia and 176 587 patients were studied with respect to brain tumors. Malignancies investigated included acute lymphoblastic leukemia, acute myeloid leukemia, myelodysplastic syndromes (MDS), leukemia excluding MDS, gliomas, meningiomas, and schwannomas. Relative risks were calculated to assess the relationship between the radiation doses expressed in mGy units and malignancy. Data were collected from a national registry and ended on December 31, 2008, at time of death, or when patients were lost to follow-up. During analysis, radiation doses were adjusted to reflect the time it typically takes to develop a malignancy. This resulted in a 2 year lag for leukemia and a 5 year lag for brain tumors.

Among the patients included in the leukemia analysis, 283 919 CT scans were completed (64% head) and 74 patients had developed leukemia on follow-up. 279 824 scans were completed for patients included in brain tumor analysis with 135 patients ultimately receiving diagnoses of brain tumors on follow-up. Significant positive associations between leukemia and CT radiation dosing ($p < 0.01$) and brain tumors and radiation ($p < 0.001$) were observed. Mean radiation dose was 51.13 mGy for patients who developed leukemia and with exposure to ≥30 mGy of radiation. Among those who received ≥30 mGy, patients were more than 3 times as likely to develop leukemia when compared to those who received <5 mGy (RR 3.18; 95%CI 1.46-6.94). Mean radiation dose for patients who received ≥50 mGy and developed brain tumors was 104.16 mGy. Those who received ≥50 mGy of radiation were at greater than 3 times the risk of developing a brain tumor when compared to those who were exposed to <5 mGy (RR 3.32; 95%CI 1.84-6.42).

Pearce MS, Salotti JA, Little MP, McHugh K, Lee C, Kim KP, et al. Radiation exposure from CT scans in childhood and subsequent risk of leukaemia and brain tumors: a retrospective cohort. The Lancet. 2012 Aug 4;380(9840):499–505.

Increased use of pediatric CT poses significant oncogenic risk

1. Between 1996 and 2010, the use of computed tomographic (CT) imaging increased 2- to 3-fold for children up to 14 years of age, with effective radiation doses per scan varying widely, but ranging up to 69.2 mSv/scan.

2. The highest average radiation doses were delivered by abdominal and pelvic CT scans, with up to a quarter of such scans providing over 20 mSv/scan. A corresponding lifetime attributable risk of solid oncogenesis was estimated at 1 tumor for every 300-390 scans at worst, varying by age, sex, and scan type.

Original Date of Publication: June 2013

Study Rundown: The expanding uses of pediatric imaging have dramatically improved modern diagnostic capabilities. With this expansion has come an increasing concern for the possibility of associated oncogenic risk due to the delivery of ionizing radiation from techniques such as CT. Children are thought to have increased risk of radiation-induced cancers due to their young age, reduced radiation attenuation secondary to smaller body sizes, and the potential for increased radiation doses due to a failure to appropriately alter scanning protocols from an adult to a pediatric paradigm. Previously, Mathews et al. estimated that the incidence of cancers due to childhood CT exposure was 24% higher in irradiated subjects than controls, with risk increases proportional to dose, and inversely proportional to age at exposure. The current study sought to retrospectively examine trends in CT use, including doses delivered to children during individual CT scans, and project an attributable carcinogenic risk of such scans in an effort to offer targeted dose reduction strategies. During the study period from 1996 to 2010, the authors found that CT use had sharply increased, doubling for children under age 5 and tripling for those aged 5-14 before peaking around 2007 and downtrending thereafter. Effective single scan doses were highly variable across sites and scanners, ranging from 0.03 to 69.2 mSv/scan, with up to a quarter of children receiving doses greater than 20 mSv/scan. The most frequently ordered scans were of the abdomen and pelvis, which also carried the highest average radiation dose and corresponding oncogenic risk, estimated at 25.8 to 33.9 cases per 10 000 scans for girls, and 13.1 to 14.8 cases per 10 000 for boys. Lifetime attributable solid cancer and leukemia risks were calculated based on individual organ dosimetry and were highest for girls and younger children. These data suggested that nearly 5000 future cancers could be attributed to pediatric CT use per year in the United States, and that a reduction of the highest quartile of doses could prevent over two fifths of such cancers.

In-Depth [retrospective cohort]: Between 1996 and 2010, this study retrospectively observed CT use patterns in children aged 15 or younger at six large health maintenance organizations (HMOs) within the HMO Research Network across the United States. Roughly 150 000 to 370 000 children were included in the study per year (50% female, 29% under 5 years of age). CT use increased steadily between 1996 and 2005, peaking at a doubling of scans for children under age 5 and a tripling of scans for children aged 5 to 14. From 2007 onward, CT utilization trended down. The most commonly ordered scans were of the head, abdomen/pelvis, thorax and spine, respectively, with abdominal/pelvic scans seeing the greatest increase in use. Effective radiation doses, on a per organ basis, were calculated using age- and sex-specific computational anatomy phantoms and the abstracted study parameters of 744 randomly selected individual scans. From these data, lifetime attributable risks of cancer were projected using multiple previously published risk models based upon data from the Life Span Study of Japanese atomic bomb survivors. Solid tumor risks increased with earlier ages at exposure, increased dose, and female gender. Using abdomen/pelvis CTs as the highest risk index scenario, 1 radiation-induced tumor was predicted for every 300-390 and 670-760 scans for girls and boys, respectively). Leukemia risks were highest for head CTs in children under age 5, at 1 case of leukemia per 5250 head CTs performed in this age group. Projection of these findings to the United States at large suggested that each year, pediatric CT imaging could conservatively be attributable to the development of 4870 future cancers. Reductions in delivered doses or scan frequency through standardized pediatric dose reduction protocols, increased use of alternative imaging modalities such as ultrasound or magnetic resonance imaging, and implementation of stricter appropriateness guidelines to reduce unnecessary scans could significantly reduce oncogenic risks. More specifically, a reduction of the highest 25% of doses delivered per scan to the median dose could prevent 43% of attributable tumors, while a 33% reduction in CTs performed would reduce cancers by an equal proportion.

Miglioretti DL, Johnson E, Williams A, Greenlee RT, Weinman S, Solberg LI, et al. The use of computed tomography in pediatrics and the associated radiation exposure and estimated cancer risk. Journal of the American Medical Association. 2013 Jun 10;167(8):700–07.

Mathews JD, Forsythe AV, Brady Z, Butler MW, Goergen SK, Byrnes GB, et al. Cancer risk in 680 000 people exposed to computed tomography scans in childhood or adolescence: data linkage study of 11 million Australians. BMJ. 2013 May 21;346:f2360.

This page left intentionally blank.

II. Screening Literature

"A fact is a simple statement that everyone believes. It is innocent, unless found guilty. A hypothesis is a novel suggestion that no one wants to believe. It is guilty, until found effective."

- Edward Teller, PhD

The NLST: CT screening reduces lung cancer mortality

1. Low-dose computed tomography (CT) screening significantly reduced lung cancer mortality when compared to screening with chest radiography.

2. Screening for lung cancer with either modality resulted in very high false positive rates.

Original Date of Publication: August 2011

Study Rundown: Prior studies have shown that lung cancer screening using chest radiography does not decrease lung cancer mortality. The use of molecular markers in screening is also under study, but currently unsuitable for clinical application. In contrast, observational studies have suggested that low-dose helical CT may be superior to chest radiography in detecting early-stage lung cancer. The National Lung Screening Trial (NLST) was a randomized, controlled study that compared 3 annual low-dose CTs with chest radiography in lung cancer screening. In summary, this study demonstrated that low-dose CT screening significantly reduced lung cancer-related mortality when compared with chest radiography. Additionally, low-dose CT screening detected more lower-stage cancers than chest radiography and low-dose CT significantly decreased all-cause mortality.

Strengths of the study include the participants' high adherence rate. Approximately 95% of participants adhered to the three rounds of screening in the low-dose CT group, while 93% adhered in the radiography group. Advancements in CT scanners since the time of the study may lead to further reductions in lung cancer mortality, though may also contribute to higher rates of false positives. The major limitations of this study are the limited follow-up and the very high false-positive rates in both the CT and radiography groups. Recently, the United States Preventive Services Task Force issued a draft statement recommending screening high-risk individuals with low-dose CT on an annual basis based on the results of the NLST trial, though there remains controversy in this area. The American Cancer Society, for example, recommends discussing screening with low-dose CT, while cautioning patients about the high likelihood of false positives and potential further investigation.

In-Depth [randomized controlled trial]: The NLST was a randomized trial that enrolled 53 454 patients. Eligible patients were between 55-74 years of age, had at least a 30 pack-year smoking history, and, if former smokers, had stopped smoking within the last 15 years. The exclusion criteria were a previous diagnosis of lung cancer, having a chest CT in the previous 18 months, hemoptysis, or unexplained weight loss in the previous year. In the end, 26 722 patients were randomized to screening through 3 annual low-dose CTs and 26 732 to 3 annual chest radiographs. Chest radiography, rather than community care, was chosen for the control group because the concomitant Pancreatic, Lung, Colorectal, and Ovarian (PLCO) cancer trial was evaluating the effect of chest radiography versus community care for lung cancer. Data analysis was conducted according to the intention-to-screen principle. For low-dose CT, any non-calcified nodule larger than 4 mm in diameter was classified as a positive finding. For chest radiography, any non-calcified nodule was classified as a positive finding. Results showed that low-dose CT was associated with a significant 20.0% relative reduction in lung cancer mortality (95%CI 6.8-26.7%, p = 0.004). Low-dose CT was also associated with significantly higher incidence of lung cancer (RR 1.13; 95%CI 1.03-1.23). All-cause mortality was significantly lower in the low-dose CT group by 6.7% (95%CI 1.2-13.6%, p = 0.02).

National Lung Screening Trial Research Team, Aberle DR, Adams AM, Berg CD, Black WC, Clapp JD, et al. Reduced lung-cancer mortality with low-dose computed tomographic screening. The New England Journal of Medicine. 2011 Aug 4;365(5):395–409.

LUNG-RADS criteria increases positive predictive value for lung cancer detection in high-risk patients

1. The American College of Radiology (ACR) developed the Lung Imaging Reporting and Data System (Lung-RADS) to standardize reporting and management of CT lung cancer screenings (Table I).

2. Retrospective application of Lung-RADS criteria, notably with a higher nodule size thresholds delineating a positive screening result, resulted in an increased positive predictive value (PPV) of lung cancer diagnosis in high-risk patients receiving CT lung screenings relative to National Lung Screening Trial (NLST) nodule size thresholds.

Original Date of Publication: May 2014

Study Rundown: Early in the progression of lung cancer symptoms are rare, but persistent cough, dyspnea, chest pain, and/or weight loss may be experienced in advanced forms of the disease. Most lung cancers are caused by exposure to tobacco smoke. Because symptoms are rare in early forms of the disease it is recommended for people at increased risk for lung cancer to undergo regular screenings. Results from the National Lung Screening Trial (NLST) indicated chest CT screenings can decrease lung cancer deaths significantly relative to screenings with chest x-rays. In addition, the NLST study indicated CT screening leads to more false positives than chest x-rays, with the false positive rate hovering at approximately 98%.

The NLST defined a positive lung CT screening result to be a nodule greater than 4 mm in diameter with no benign calcification patterns. Because increasing the threshold to diagnose a lesion as cancerous can theoretically decrease the false positive rate but also decrease the sensitivity of the screening procedure, questions have been raised about changing the thresholds for positive cancer diagnosis. Additionally, management of patients with positive screening results has not been truly standardized. Lung-RADS has sought to address these issues by increasing the thresholds for a positive screening test and providing management guidelines on how to proceed after screening. Retrospective studies by McKee and colleagues and Pinsky and colleagues indicate the PPV of CT screenings of high-risk patients can be raised significantly with small or no decreases in sensitivity.

In-Depth [retrospective cohorts]: Pinsky and colleagues applied the Lung-RADS criteria to published data from the NLST. Patients aged 55-74 who smoked for 30+ pack-years and still smoked or had quit in the last 15 years were recruited at 33 US institutions for the study (n=26 455). Patient and nodule level information was available for analysis. To assess Lung-RADS, nodules were reclassified using categories ranging from 1 (negative screening) to 4 (suspicious), with Category 4 having various subcategories. Classification of nodules using Lung-RADS accounts for nodule size, attenuation, and nodule growth in follow-up screenings. Positive results, as well as follow-up and management guidelines, are detailed in Table I. The patient's screening category is based off the nodule with the highest Lung-RADS score. Lung cancer was considered present at a given screening if the diagnosis was made within 1 year of screening or before the next screening. When applying Lung-RADS criteria to baseline and follow-up screenings false-positive rates and sensitivity were significantly lower.

McKee and colleagues also retrospectively assessed application of Lung-RADS criteria to CT lung cancer screenings originally assessed using National Comprehensive Cancer Network (NCCN) criteria. Patients were assessed at a single center and had to be at high-risk for lung cancer (as defined by NCCN), asymptomatic, have physician orders for CT lung screening, been cancer free the previous 5+ years, and not have metastatic disease (n=2180). Reclassification of nodules to benign using Lung-RADS occurred in 17% (370/2180) of patients, decreasing positive test rates from 27.6% using NCCN criteria to 10.6%. No patients diagnosed with lung cancer following screening had their nodules reclassified to benign. The PPV of baseline CT screening increased from 6.9% to 17.3%. Of 29 patients diagnosed with lung cancer on follow-up, 86.3% (25/29) were classified as Category 4.

ACR. Lung CT Screening Reporting and Data System (Lung-RADS™) - American College of Radiology [Internet]. 2014. Available from: http://www.acr.org/Quality-Safety/Resources/LungRADS.

Additional Review:

Pinsky P, Gierada D, Black W, Munden R, Nath H, Aberle D, Kazerooni E. Performance of Lung-RADS in the National Lung Screening Trial. Annals of Internal Medicine. 2015;162(7):485.

Lung-RADS Framework

Category	Descriptor	Findings	Management
0	**Incomplete**	- Prior chest CT examination(s) in the process of being located - Part or all of the lungs cannot be evaluated	Additional lung cancer screening CT images and/or comparison to prior chest CT examinations is needed
1	**Negative:** No nodules and definitely benign nodules	- No lung nodules - Nodule(s) with specific calcification patterns: complete, popcorn, central, concentric rings and fat containing nodules	Continue annual screening with LDCT in 12 months
2	**Benign Appearance or Behavior:** Nodules with a very low likelihood of becoming a clinically active cancer due to size or lack of growth	- Solids nodule(s): o <6 mm o New <4 mm - Part solid nodule(s): o <6 mm total diameter on baseline screening - Nonsolid nodule(s) (GGN): o <20 mm OR o ≥20 mm and unchanged or slowly growing - Category 3 or 4 nodules unchanged for ≥3 months	Continue annual screening with LDCT in 12 months
3	**Probably Benign:** Probably benign finding(s) - short term follow up suggested; includes nodules with a low likelihood of becoming a clinically active cancer	- Solid nodule(s): o ≥6 to <8 mm at basclinc OR o New 4 mm to <6 mm - Part solid nodule(s) o ≥6 mm total diameter with solid component <6 mm OR o New <6 mm in diameter - Nonsolid nodule(s) (GGNs) ≥20 mm on baseline CT or new	6 month LDCT

4A	**Suspicious:** Findings for which additional diagnostic testing and/or tissue sampling is recommended	- Solid nodule(s): o ≥8 to <15 mm at baseline OR o Growing <8 mm OR o New 6 to <8 mm	3 month LDCT; PET/CT may be used when there is a ≥8 mm solid component
		- Part solid nodule(s): o ≥6 mm with solid component ≥6 to <8 mm OR o With a new or growing <4 mm solid component	
		- Endobronchial nodule	
4B		- Solid nodule(s): o ≥15 mm OR o New or growing and ≥8 mm	Chest CT with or without contrast, PET/CT and/or tissue sampling depending on the probability of malignancy and comorbidities. PET/CT may be used when there is a ≥8 mm solid component.
		- Part solid nodule(s) with: o A solid component ≥8 mm OR o A new or growing ≥4 mm solid component	
4X		- Category 3 or 4 nodules with additional features or imaging findings that increases the suspicion of malignancy	
S	**Significant:** Clinically significant or potentially clinically significant findings (non lung cancer)	- Modifier: may add on to category 0-4 coding	As appropriate to specific finding
C	**Prior Lung Cancer**	- Modifier: may add on to category 0-4 coding	-

Table I. Lung-RADS final assessment categories. LDCT = Low Dose CT. GGN = Ground Glass Nodule. Table compiled using information from https://www.acr.org/-/media/ACR/Files/RADS/Lung-RADS/LungRADS_AssessmentCategories.pdf

BI-RADS identifies mammography features with high positive predictive values for carcinoma

Breast cancer is the second leading cause of cancer death in women. Given that many early breast cancers are asymptomatic and elude detection by physical exam, mammography was developed as a screening tool to uncover breast cancers at an earlier stage, thereby improving prognosis. The American Cancer Society currently recommends that women of average breast cancer risk begin obtaining annual screening mammograms between the ages of 40 and 45 depending on preference, with the option to switch to biennial screening after age 55. Modified screening protocols starting at an earlier age are employed in patients with higher risk on the basis of family history or genetic risk modifiers.

Mammograms can reveal a spectrum of findings, some of which prompt suspicion for malignancy but many of which are benign. The growth of mammography in the 1980s resulted in a compelling need to craft a standardized reporting system for describing these findings and translating them into management recommendations. In response, the American College of Radiology (ACR) developed the Breast Imaging-Reporting and Data System (BI-RADS) system, which comprises a lexicon for describing mammographic findings, a structure for mammography reports, a set of final assessment categories with management guidelines, and technical recommendations for performing mammographic studies. The first edition of BI-RADS was released in 1993 with the intent of allowing periodic updates as new data and clinical experience emerged. Subsequent iterations built upon the original BI-RADS structure, with the fourth edition in 2003 introducing analogous reporting constructs for breast ultrasound and breast MRI. Currently, BI-RADS is in its fifth edition (released in 2013) and remains the standard reporting paradigm in breast imaging. **Please see Tables I-III for the current BI-RADS classification and lexicon.**

As an early effort to characterize the performance of the first edition of BI-RADS and inform future modification of the reporting terminology, the following study by Liberman et al. evaluated the positive predictive value (PPV) of the various BI-RADS terms used for mammographic interpretation. Findings revealed that several features pertaining to masses (spiculated margins, irregular shape) and calcifications (linear morphology, segmental or linear distribution) were highly associated with malignancy, demonstrating positive predictive values ranging from 68-81%.

1. Lesions observed in mammography with spiculated margins, linear calcification morphology, irregular shape, segmental calcification distribution, or linear calcification distributions have high PPVs for breast malignancy (81%, 81%, 73%, 74%, 68%, respectively).

2. Using the BI-RADS framework and lexicon (Tables I-III), radiologists had very comparable PPVs for detecting carcinoma in lesions categorized as a 4 or 5.

Original Date of Publication: July 1998

Study Rundown: Seeking to better standardize characterization and reporting of mammography readings, the ACR developed BI-RADS nomenclature. This study sought to evaluate the positive predictive value of the various descriptive terms BI-RADS offers for mammogram interpretation. Results showed that among lesions that would typically be followed up by physicians, several lesional features were highly associated with cancerous biopsies, with positive predictive values for carcinoma ranging from 68-81%. Utilization of BI-RADS terminology also showed different radiologists characterized lesions into various final assessment categories describing the suspicion of cancerous lesions at statistically similar rates.

In-Depth [prospective cohort]: Patients at Memorial-Sloan Kettering with impalpable breast lesions seen upon initial mammographic interpretation were referred for surgical tissue biopsy. Prior to surgery, 1 of 5 academic radiologists evaluated the mammographic lesion images. Lesions that had already undergone a prior biopsy were excluded from the study and image interpretation. In total, 492 lesions from 466 women (median age 52, range 27-92) were included in the study, with 73 (16%) of the women having had breast cancer previously. Lesions were characterized using BI-RADS terminology describing mass margins and shape, and calcification morphology and distribution. The most worrisome descriptor in the radiologist's interpretation was used to give the lesion a final classification on a scale of 1 (normal mammography) to 5 (highly suggestive of malignancy).

Carcinoma was confirmed in 225 (46%) of the lesions. Within subcategories of lesions, 50% (79/158) of noncalcified masses, 86% (12/14) of calcified masses, and 42% (134/320) of calcifications without mass were carcinomas. BI-RADS final assessments by reading radiologists placed 26% (129/492) of lesions in category 5, 72% (355/492) in category 4, and 2% (8/492) in category 3.

Carcinoma was confirmed in 81% (105/129) of category 5, 34% (120/355) of category 4, and 0% (0/8) of category 3 lesions. Amongst the BI-RADS features used to assign final assessment grades to lesions, high positive predictive values were found in 5 of them: spiculated margins (81%), linear calcification morphology (81%), irregular shape (73%), segmental calcification distribution (74%), or linear calcification distribution (68%).

Liberman L, Abramson A, Squires F, Glassman J, Morris E, Dershaw D. The breast imaging reporting and data system: positive predictive value of mammographic features and final assessment categories. American Journal of Roentgenology*. 1998;171(1):35-40.*

Additional Review:

ACR. ACR BI-RADS® Atlas - American College of Radiology [Internet]. 2016. Available from: http://www.acr.org/Quality-Safety/Resources/BIRADS.

BI-RADS Framework			
Category	**Descriptor**	**Management**	**Cancer Probability**
0	Incomplete – Need additional imaging evaluation and/or prior mammograms for comparison	Further imaging needed	N/A
1	Negative	Routine screening	0%
2	Benign	Routine screening	0%
3	Probably benign	Short interval follow-up	<2%
4	Suspicious	Consider biopsy	4a. Low suspicion (≥2 to ≤10%) 95% 4b. Moderate suspicion (>10 to ≤50%) 4c. High suspicion (>50% to <95%)
5	Highly suggestive of malignancy	Biopsy or surgery	≥95%
6	Known biopsy-proven malignancy	Appropriate action (i.e., surgery)	N/A

Table I. BI-RADS classification.
Table compiled using information from www.acr.org/Quality-Safety/Resources/BIRADS.

<table>
<tr><th colspan="4">BI-RADS 5th Edition Mammography Lexicon</th></tr>
<tr><td>Breast composition</td><td colspan="3">a. Entirely fatty
b. Scattered areas of fibroglandular density
c. Heterogeneously dense, which may obscure masses
d. Extremely dense, which lowers sensitivity</td></tr>
<tr><td rowspan="3">Mass</td><td>shape</td><td colspan="2">oval / round / irregular</td></tr>
<tr><td>margin</td><td colspan="2">circumscribed / obscured / microlobulated / indistinct / spiculated</td></tr>
<tr><td>density</td><td colspan="2">fat / low / equal / high</td></tr>
<tr><td>Asymmetry</td><td colspan="3">asymmetry / global / focal / developing</td></tr>
<tr><td>Architectural distortion</td><td colspan="3">Distorted parenchyma with no visible mass</td></tr>
<tr><td rowspan="3">Calcifications</td><td rowspan="2">morphology</td><td>typically benign</td><td>skin / vascular / coarse "popcorn like" / large rod-like / round / rim / dystrophic / milk of calcium / suture</td></tr>
<tr><td>suspicious</td><td>amorphous / coarse heterogenous / fine pleiomorphic / fine linear or fine linear branching</td></tr>
<tr><td>distribution</td><td colspan="2">diffuse / regional / grouped / linear / segmental</td></tr>
<tr><td>Associated features</td><td colspan="3">skin retraction / nipple retraction / skin thickening / trabecular thickening / axillary adenopathy / architectural distortion / calcifications</td></tr>
<tr><td>Location</td><td colspan="3">laterality / quadrant and clock face / depth / distance from the nipple</td></tr>
</table>

Table II. Updated BI-RADS fifth Edition (2013) mammography lexicon. Table compiled using information from www.acr.org/Quality-Safety/Resources/BIRADS.

BI-RADS 5th Edition Ultrasound Lexicon		
Tissue composition (screening only)	a. homogenous - fat b. homogenous - fibroglandular c. heterogenous	
Mass	shape	oval / round / irregular
	margin	a. circumscribed b. not circumscribed (indistinct, angular, microlobulated, spiculated)
	orientation	parallel / not parallel
	echo pattern	anechoic / hyperechoic / complex cystic and solid / isoechoic / heterogenous
	posterior features	no features / enhancement / shadowing / combined pattern
Calcifications	in mass / outside mass / intraductal	
Associated features	architectural distortion / duct changes / skin changes (thickening, retraction) / edema / vascularity (absent, internal, rim) / elasticity (soft, intermediate, hard)	
Special cases	simple cyst / clustered microcysts / complicated cyst / mass in or on skin / foreign body including implants / intramammary or axillary lymph nodes / AVMs / Mondor disease / postsurgical fluid collection / fat necrosis	

Table III. Updated BI-RADS fifth Edition (2013) ultrasound lexicon. Table compiled using information from www.acr.org/Quality-Safety/Resources/BIRADS.

Breast MRI most sensitive screening modality in high-risk patients

1. Among patients with a familial or genetic predisposition to the development of breast cancer, magnetic resonance imaging (MRI) of the breast was significantly more sensitive than either clinical exam or mammography for the detection of invasive breast cancer.

2. Invasive breast cancers detected by MRI were more frequently less than one centimeter in diameter and displayed a lower incidence of axillary nodal metastases or micrometastases than those detected by mammography or clinical breast exam.

Original Date of Publication: July 2004

Study Rundown: Breast cancer screening for women aged 50 to 70 has been shown to significantly reduce cancer-related mortality. However, for women with a strong family history of early breast cancer or known germline oncogenic mutations such as the *BRCA1* or *BRCA2* mutations, screening at an earlier age may be warranted due to their high lifetime cancer risk. Screening of the general population at younger ages has been of unclear value due to increased breast density among premenopausal women potentially reducing the sensitivity of mammography. Among those with genetic predispositions to breast cancer, mammography has been further limited, demonstrating a low sensitivity for cancer detection due in part to rapid tumor growth and an increased incidence of atypical historadiological characteristics of the tumors in these women. Contrast-enhanced breast MRI had been suggested as an alternative screening modality for high-risk women given its high sensitivity and the relative indifference of the modality to breast density. In the referenced article, yearly mammography and serial clinical breast examinations were prospectively compared to yearly screening breast MRI in younger women with an established predisposition to breast cancer. In nearly 3 years of screening high-risk women with a mean age of 40 years, contrast-enhanced breast MRI was by far the most sensitive modality at 79.5%, performing significantly better than either mammography or clinical breast exam at 33.3% and 17.9%, respectively. However, the specificity and positive predictive value of MRI was the lowest of the three methods at 89.8% and 7.1%, as compared to mammography at 95.0% and 8.0%, respectively. Notably, tumors detected by breast MRI were significantly more likely to be of lower stage, with more tumors found at sizes less than 10 mm in diameter, and fewer tumors with micrometastases or axillary nodal metastases, suggesting earlier detection in the natural course of the disease. No differences in disease-free or overall survival could be determined as no mortalities were recorded during the course of the study. These findings demonstrated that MRI had significantly better overall discriminating capacity than either mammography or clinical breast exam in screening women at high-risk for breast cancer.

In-Depth [prospective cohort]: This prospective trial enrolled 1909 women (mean age 40 years; range 19-72 years, 75% premenopausal) at multiple centers across Europe who were known to be at high risk for breast cancer (greater than 15% lifetime risk) due either to a strong family history of early breast cancer or known genetic mutation. Women were excluded from the study if they had symptoms suggestive of current breast cancer or a personal history of breast cancer. All subjects were screened by twice yearly clinical breast exam and yearly mammography and contrast-enhanced breast MRI over a median follow-up period of 2.9 years (mean 2.7, range 0.1-3.9 years). Results from each modality were blinded such that no examination could influence another. Radiologic studies were scored on the BI-RADS system, with the threshold for positivity set to category 3 ("probably benign or uncertain result") for both statistical analysis and further investigation by ultrasonography, fine-needle aspiration, or biopsy as necessary. Results of these further investigations were used to diagnose a tumor as benign or malignant, and formed the basis for subsequent determinations of specificity and positive predictive value for each screening modality. The overall sensitivity of MRI for the detection of invasive breast cancers (excluding ductal carcinoma in situ) among high-risk women was 79.5% using BI-RADS 3 or higher as the cutoff for positivity, as compared to 17.9% for clinical breast exam and 33.3% for mammography. The specificity of clinical examination was the highest at 98.1%, while mammography and breast MRI were 95.0% and 89.8%, respectively. The positive predictive value of MRI was 7.1% as compared to 9.6% for clinical exam and 8.0% for mammography. Based on the area under the receiver operator curves for both MRI and mammography, MRI showed a significantly better discriminating capacity than mammography (Difference in AUC 0.141, 95%CI 0.020-0.262; $p < 0.05$). Tumors detected by MRI were generally of a lower stage than those detected by alternative methods, with 43.2% found at a diameter of less than 10 mm, versus only 12.5% and 14.0% in each respective average risk control group ($p < 0.001$ and $p = 0.04$). Additionally, the incidence of either positive axillary lymph node metastases or micrometastases was 21.4% as compared to 52.4% and 56.4% in each control group ($p < 0.001$ and $p = 0.001$, respectively.) During the median 2.9 years of follow up, none of the patients with breast cancer died, therefore no difference of disease-free or overall survival could be assessed.

Kriege M, Brekelmans CT, Boetes C, Besnard PE, Zonderland HM, Obdeijn IM, et al. Efficacy of MRI and Mammography for Breast-Cancer Screening in Women with a Familial or Genetic Predisposition. The New England Journal of Medicine. 2004 Jul 29;351(5):427–37.

Combination mammography and breast tomosynthesis improves breast cancer screening

1. The addition of breast tomosynthesis to digital mammography in breast cancer screening improved lesion conspicuity, thereby significantly increasing the rate of cancer detection and the overall positive predictive value of screening.

2. The rate of patient recall for further workup of a positive screen was significantly reduced with the addition of tomosynthesis.

Original Date of Publication: June 2014

Study Rundown: Breast cancer screening generally, with a few notable exceptions, entails yearly mammography and clinical breast exam for women aged 50-70 years, among whom it has been shown to reduce mortality. However, mammography alone suffers from a limited positive predictive value, with an excess of false-positive results believed to be due to overlapping breast tissue. Breast tomosynthesis (BT) was developed to offset this limitation. By acquiring multiple low-dose images of the breast at focal planes of varying depth and reconstructing a single image or depth stacked series of images, BT reduces the "noise" of overlapping densities within the breast to more easily highlight true abnormalities. As imaging technology has progressed with large-field, fast-reading detectors, BT has now become feasible in routine practice, and the referenced study sought to examine how large-scale combination of mammography and BT compares to mammography alone in improving upon the specificity of breast cancer screening. In a retrospective review of nearly a half million screening examinations performed before and after the introduction of combined mammography and BT in routine practice, the combination technique significantly increased the positive predictive value of a positive screening examination from 4.3% to 6.4%, and of a subsequent biopsy from 24.2% to 29.2%. This improvement was reflected in an increase in the cancer detection rate at screening from 4.2 by mammography alone to 5.4 per 1000 examinations by the combined method. Additionally, the combination of mammography and BT reduced the overall recall rate, or the proportion of patients in whom a positive screen necessitated further workup, from 107 to 91 per 1000 examinations. Together, these findings suggested that the addition of BT to routine breast cancer screening may improve screening specificity, thereby reducing unnecessary interventions due to false-positive results. However, a direct determination of sensitivity and specificity could not be calculated as the dataset did not include patient-level information on the occurrence of interval cancers. The study was additionally limited by its retrospective nature and inherent lack of randomization, introducing the potential for selection bias and differences in baseline patient characteristics to influence the results obtained.

In-Depth [retrospective cohort]: This retrospective trial was conducted at 13 separate sites over two separate periods, one prior to the introduction of BT at each institution (one year in duration), and the other following the start of standard screening with combined digital mammography and BT (average duration of 17 months). Notably, only two sites were able to replace all equipment with tomography capable devices at once, while others maintained a hybrid environment in which mammography alone was still used after the transition. A total of 454 850 screening examinations were included in the primary analysis, read by 139 radiologists across all sites, with 61.8% performed during the first period (mammography alone), and 38.2% performed during the second period (mammography + BT). Comparing those studies performed prior to the introduction of BT to mammographic screening, a specific set of metrics was tabulated to compare the efficacy of mammography with and without BT: The patient recall rate, or proportion of patients in whom a positive screen necessitated additional imaging; the cancer detection rate, or proportion of patients in whom a positive screen detected a true cancer, and the positive predictive value for both patient recall and for biopsies performed as a result of a screening examination. For mammography alone, the rate of patient recall was 107 per 1000 screens as compared to 91 per 1000 screens for mammography + BT, resulting in a decrease in the recall rate of -16 (95%CI -18 to -14; $p < 0.001$) per 1000 screens. The difference in biopsy rate between mammography without and with BT was +1.3 (95%CI 0.4-2.1; $p = 0.004$) per 1000 screens. The overall cancer detection rate (n=815 invasive cancers, n=392 ductal carcinoma in situ) for mammography alone was 4.2 per 1000 screens, while it increased to 5.4 per 1000 screens with the addition of tomography, resulting in an increase of 1.2 (95%CI 0.8-1.6; $p < 0.001$) per 1000 screens. When considering invasive cancers alone, the net increase in cancer detection rate was unchanged. The PPV for recall for mammography alone was 4.3% versus 6.4% with the addition of BT, for an overall increase of 2.1% (95%CI 1.7-2.5% $p < 0.001$), while for biopsy, the net increase in PPV was 5.0% (95%CI 3.0-7.0%; $p < 0.001$). A secondary analysis was performed using examinations the second period alone, comparing mammograms performed without BT to those performed with BT in an effort to address the potential for selection bias to affect the results given the hybrid nature of the transition at many sites. A statistically significant improvement in cancer detection with mammography + BT was found ($p < 0.001$), consistent with those findings from the primary analysis.

Friedewald SM, Rafferty EA, Rose SL, Durand MA, Plecha DM, Greenberg JS, et al. Breast Cancer Screening Using Tomosynthesis in Combination With Digital Mammography. The Journal of The American Medical Association. 2014 Jun 25;311(24):2499–2507.

LI-RADS outlines standards for liver imaging studies assessing HCC

1. The American College of Radiology (ACR) created the Liver Imaging Reporting and Data System (LI-RADS) to standardize interpretation and reporting of liver imaging studies assessing risk for hepatocellular carcinoma (HCC).

2. Utilization of LI-RADS categories can aid in patient management decisions by suggesting diagnostic and/or treatment options.

Original Date of Publication: March 2011

Study Rundown: Chronic liver disease (CLD) and cirrhosis are risk factors for HCC, the third leading cause of cancer-related death worldwide. With these factors contributing towards development of the disease, HCC can affect a wide range of communities and counties. Early stage HCC is often asymptomatic and detection earlier is associated with better outcomes when medical treatment is offered, making screening of patients at high risk for HCC a key intervention. Screening evaluations can be completed using a variety of methods, with computed tomography (CT) or magnetic resonance imaging (MRI) being the most common.

LI-RADS, originally published in 2011 and continually updated, provides a standardized algorithmic framework for assessing HCC risk via CT or MRI. In addition to reducing variability in radiologist reporting, the framework can help clinicians by providing recommendations for how to follow-up lesions with further imaging studies, biopsies, and/or treatment. Though this system provides a standardized mechanism for lesion categorization, few prospective studies have been performed assessing how patients are differentially managed when assigned differing risk categories.

In-Depth: LI-RADS was developed by a panel of radiologists, with additional contribution from hepatologists, liver surgeons, and pathologists. The first iteration was launched in 2011 and has been updated continually since. LI-RADS provides standardized terminology for interpreting hepatic lesions and categorizing them according to their risk of HCC based on image characteristics (Table I). Categorization ranges from "Definitely Benign" (LR-

1) to "Definitely HCC" (LR-5). Categorization of lesions as "Probably Benign" (LR-2), "Intermediate Probability of HCC" (LR-3), and "Probably HCC" (LR-4) are based on 4 major image factors defined by Mitchell and colleagues including: arterial phase hyperenhancement; washout appearance following hyperenhancement; capsule appearance; and threshold growth compared with previous imaging. If there is uncertainty as to a categorization between LR-2 and LR-4, various defined ancillary image features may be used (Table 2). Additionally, there are categories for probable malignancy other than HCC (LR-M), previously treated HCC (LR5-T), and tumor within a vein (LR-5V).

Mitchell DG, Bruix J, Sherman M, Sirlin CB. LI-RADS (Liver Imaging Reporting and Data System): Summary, discussion, and consensus of the LI-RADS Management Working Group and future directions. Hepatology. 2015 Mar 1;61(3):1056–65.

Additional Review:

ACR. Archive - LI-RADS [Internet]. 2011. Available from: http://www.acr.org/Quality-Safety/Resources/LIRADS/Archive.

Purysko AS, Remer EM, Coppa CP, Leão Filho HM, Thupili CR, Veniero JC. LI-RADS: A Case-based Review of the New Categorization of Liver Findings in Patients with End-Stage Liver Disease. RadioGraphics. 2012 Nov 1;32(7):1977–95.

LI-RADS Framework

Category	Probability of HCC	Imaging Features	Management
LR-1	Definitely benign	• Diagnostic features for a benign entity OR • Lesion resolves without treatment	• Continue standard surveillance
LR-2	Probably benign	• Suggestive, but not diagnostic, features for a benign entity	• Continue standard surveillance • If >1 cm, consider accelerated follow-up, alternative imaging or multidisciplinary discussion
LR-3	Intermediate probability of HCC	• Mass HYPERenhancing in the arterial phase with NO WCT • Mass HYPO- or ISOenhancing in the arterial phase: o <20 mm with ≤1 of WCT o ≥20 mm with NO WCT	• Variable • At a minimum accelerated follow-up, consider alternative imaging or multidisciplinary discussion
LR-4	Probably HCC	• Mass HYPERenhancing in the arterial phase: o <10 mm with ≥1 of WCT o 10-19 mm with 1 of WCT o ≥20 mm with NO WCT • Mass HYPO- or ISOenhancing in the arterial phase: o <20 mm with ≥2 of WCT o ≥20 mm with ≥1 of WCT	• Variable • Alternative imaging (if distinct advantage) and/or multidisciplinary discussion
LR-5	Definitely HCC	• Mass HYPERenhancing in the arterial phase: o 10-19 mm with ≥2 of WCT o ≥20 mm with ≥1 of WCT	• Multidisciplinary discussion

LR-5V	Tumor in vein	• Definite enhancing soft tissue in vein		• Multidisciplinary discussion • Contraindication to liver transplant
LR-M	Probable malignancy, but non-specific for HCC	*Favor other malignancy* • Arterial rim HYPERenhancement • Central delayed phase enhancement • Concentric enhancement • Peripheral washout • Hepatic retraction • Biliary obstruction greater than expected for size • Targetoid on DWI or hepatobiliary phase	*Favor HCC* • Diffuse arterial HYPERenhancement • Delayed washout • Capsule • Distinct rim • Intralesional fat • Diffuse T1 HYPERintensity • Tumor in vein • Nodule-in-nodule • Mosaic architecture • Spontaneous hemorrhage	• Variable, may include follow-up, alternative imaging, biopsy, treatment, and/or multidisciplinary discussion

Table I. LI-RADS framework. WCT = Washout, Capsule, and/or Threshold Growth.
NOTE: Alternative imaging is typically considered if there is a distinct advantage to the alternative modality.
Table compiled using information from Mitchell et al. and http://www.acr.org/Quality-Safety/Resources/LIRADS

Ancillary Features: LI-RADS Framework	
Favor Benignity	**Favor Malignancy**
- Homogenous T2 HYPERintensity - Homogenous T2 or T2* HYPOintensity - Hepatobiliary phase ISOintensity - No vessel distortion - Stable or reduced diameter on follow-up scans	- Mild-moderate T2 HYPERintensity - Diffusion restriction - Hepatobiliary/transitional phase HYPOintensity - Iron/fat sparing - Blood products - Diameter increase less than threshold - Favoring HCC specifically: o Distinct rim o Corona enhancement o Mosaic architecture o Nodule-in-nodule o Intralesional fat

Table II. Ancillary Features - LI-RADS Framework. Presence of these features may be used, with caution, to downgrade or upgrade the LR category by one or more levels, up to a maximum of LR-4. Absence of one or more features should not be used to upgrade or downgrade categories.
Table compiled using information from Mitchell et al. and http://www.acr.org/Quality-Safety/Resources/LIRADS

The PROMISE Trial: Coronary CT angiography not superior to functional testing in cardiac risk management

1. Computed tomographic coronary angiography (CTCA) as the initial diagnostic test for patients at intermediate risk of coronary artery disease (CAD) was not superior to functional cardiac testing with regard to all-cause mortality or major cardiovascular events over a 2-year period.

2. Patients in the CTCA group underwent significantly more cardiac catheterizations (though with fewer procedures revealing no CAD) and subsequently had an increased rate of coronary revascularization than those in the functional testing arm.

Original Date of Publication: April 2015

Study Rundown: Patients with suspected CAD, such as those with new-onset stable angina or at least one major cardiac risk factor, require diagnostic testing to determine both their burden of disease and the appropriateness of medical or surgical intervention in cardiac risk mitigation. Noninvasive testing for CAD is indicated for such intermediate-risk, ambulatory patients and has historically involved a functional test, such as a stress electro- or echocardiogram or a nuclear stress test, any of which can reveal indirect evidence of CAD if reversible ischemia is present. However, CTCA has emerged as a viable alternative to functional testing with a theoretically increased specificity given that it provides a direct anatomical assessment. It has even been proposed that CTCA may reveal nonobstructive but prognostically significant coronary lesions. The Prospective Multicenter Imaging Study for Evaluation of Chest Pain (PROMISE) randomized outpatients with new onset, stable chest pain or with at least one major cardiac risk factor to either CTCA or functional testing for CAD in an effort to determine if noninvasive anatomical testing might improve cardiac outcomes over functional testing. Over the 2-year follow-up period from initial randomization, no significant differences were found in all-cause mortality or major cardiovascular events between the two groups, though patients in the CTCA group underwent an increased rate of cardiac catheterization and subsequent surgical or percutaneous coronary revascularization. Notably, the study was not designed or powered to assess, given its relatively short length of follow-up, if the observed increased rate of catheterization and revascularization might have affected long-term outcomes. Within this limitation, PROMISE established that CTCA is not superior to standard functional cardiac testing in the initial workup of patients at intermediate risk of CAD. However, future trials are necessary to determine if the increased rate of revascularization observed within the CTCA group may yield a longitudinal mortality benefit.

In-Depth [randomized controlled trial]: A total of 10 003 outpatients (mean age 60±8.3 years, 52.7% women) presenting primarily with new onset, stable chest pain without a prior diagnosis of CAD were enrolled at several major medical centers across the United States. Patients were randomized to either undergo CTCA or functional cardiac testing for the non-urgent, non-invasive workup of suspected CAD, and were followed for a median period of 25 months. Functional tests utilized in the control arm of the trial included nuclear stress testing (67.5%), stress echocardiography (22.4%), and exercise electrocardiography (10.2%). The primary endpoints of the trial were all-cause mortality or major cardiovascular events (including complications from diagnostic or therapeutic cardiovascular procedures), while secondary endpoints included invasive cardiac catheterizations, particularly those that did not reveal CAD, and cumulative radiation exposure. Median cumulative radiation exposure was lower per patient in the CTCA group than the functional testing group (10.0 mSv versus 11.3 mSv; $p < 0.001$). The bulk of per patient exposure occurred secondary to nuclear stress testing, though overall exposure was greater within the CTCA group as 32.6% of patients in the functional testing group had no radiation exposure. The study was powered at 90% confidence to detect a 20% relative reduction in the primary endpoint between groups assuming an overall event rate of 8% at 2.5 years post-randomization. The true observed overall event rate was 3.1% for mortality or major cardiovascular events, with no significant difference between the CTCA group (3.3%) and the functional testing group (3.0%; adjusted hazard ratio 1.04; 95%CI 0.83-1.29; $p = 0.075$) over the median 25-month follow-up period. A similar rate of positive initial tests was observed between the two groups, with 10.7% of initial CTCAs and 11.7% of functional tests interpreted as positive. In the 90 days following randomization, 12.2% of patients in the CTCA group underwent cardiac catheterization as opposed to only 8.1% of the functional testing group, but catheterizations performed in the CTCA group significantly more likely to be positive (72.1% versus 52.5%; $p = 0.02$). Additionally, revascularization (either surgical or percutaneous) was significantly more commonly performed within the CTCA group, occurring in 6.2% of patients as compared to 3.2% in the functional testing group ($p < 0.001$). However, revascularization was not a trial end point, and the study was not adequately powered to assess the effect of this difference on long-term cardiovascular outcomes.

Douglas PS, Hoffmann U, Patel MR, Mark DB, Al-Khalidi HR, Cavanaugh B, et al. Outcomes of anatomical versus functional testing for coronary artery disease. The New England Journal of Medicine. 2015 Apr 2;372(14):1291–1300.

OPTN and UNOS update policy regarding hepatocellular carcinoma

1. Administrators overseeing the national liver transplantation network approved new policy to standardize radiologic imaging criteria for patients with hepatocellular carcinoma (HCC) to qualify for exemption points.

2. This new policy recommends various technical and procedural standards for CT and MR imaging, diagnosis, and classification criteria of HCC. It also seeks to standardize reporting requirements of HCC assessment to transplant networks.

Original Date of Publication: February 2013

Study Rundown: In the United States today, there are approximately three times more patients awaiting liver transplants than those who actually receive a liver. In order to distribute livers to patients determined to be most in need, the Organ Procurement and Transplantation Network (OPTN) and United Network for Organ Sharing (UNOS) set policy in 2002 giving priority to patients most ill and most likely to benefit from transplantation. Patients with early stage HCC have a very good prognosis if able to receive a transplant. Therefore, the 2002 OPTN policy was designed to be favorable to patients reported to have early stage HCC and gave exemption points to early-stage HCC patients moving them higher on the Model for End-Stage Liver Disease (MELD) scale of 6 (less ill) to 40 (gravely ill) used to guide which patients received livers (See "The MELD" summarized in *Section IV. Interface Literature*). However, the 2002 OPTN/UNOS policy had little structure guiding how HCCs should be diagnosed and reported to the networks. Assessment of UNOS data in 2006 indicated radiologic and pathologic assessment of HCCs only matched for 44.1% of cases. This prompted interest in creating new policy that would enhance imaging accuracy, diagnosis, and reporting of HCC to the transplant networks in order to better distribute liver transplants to HCC patients most likely to benefit.

The new liver allocation policy was approved by OPTN/UNOS in 2011. This policy outlines various technological and procedural standards for imaging, classifying, and reporting HCC studies to OPTN. Under the OPTN classification system there are two broad categories of classes, Class 0 and class 5. Class 0 imaging studies are not of sufficient standard to qualify for exception points, and Class 5 studies may qualify for exemption points. Based on characteristics of the tumor upon imaging, the HCC may be reported as Class 5A, 5A-g, 5B, 5T, or 5X, each of which may change the number of exemption points a patient may receive and change their likelihood of receiving a liver transplant.

In-Depth [policy update]: To increase the likelihood that patients with early-stage HCC receive a liver transplant, as their post transplant survival rates are high but current severity of illness is relatively low, these patients are given exception points on OPTN/UNOS transplant lists. New OPTN/UNOS recommendations aim to verify that patients receiving exemption points do indeed have early-stage HCC and outline technological and procedural standards to be met for imaging studies. Such standards include type of CT or MR scanner and contrast to be used. If a liver imaging study reported to OPTN/UNOS does not meet these recommended specifications, it is assigned as Class 0 and no exemption points can be applied. For Class 0 studies it is recommended that the imaging study be redone meeting stated standards.

If the imaging study meets these standards, it is Class 5 and further categorized. If the nodule in question is 1-2 cm in diameter and meets qualitative imaging criteria for HCC it is Class 5A. If a nodule appears arterially hyperenhanced, is at least 10 mm in diameter at diagnosis, and has grown 50+% in diameter over a period of 6 months or less is Class 5A-g. A patient having 2-3 Class 5A or 5A-g lesions would qualify them for exemption points. Arterially enhanced 2-5 cm nodules with at least one of two venous phase features (washout or pseudocapsule), or arterially enhanced 2-5 cm nodules displaying 50+% growth in diameter over a period of 6 months or less is Class 5B. Exemption points may be individually requested for Class 5B nodules. Arterially enhanced 5+cm nodules with at least one of two venous features is Class 5X and typically not eligible for liver transplant. Nodules categorized as Class 5 or confirmed as HCC upon biopsy which were subsequently treated are Class 5T. Class 5T nodules may receive exemption points based on the prior treatment and size. Reports to OPTN seeking exemption points for HCC must use the described classification system. A summary at the end of the report listing number, location, and size of nodules is strongly encouraged.

Wald C, Russo M, Heimbach J, Hussain H, Pomfret E, Bruix J. New OPTN/UNOS Policy for Liver Transplant Allocation: Standardization of Liver Imaging, Diagnosis, Classification, and Reporting of Hepatocellular Carcinoma. Radiology. 2013;266(2):376-382.

Detection of advanced colorectal neoplasia by CT colonography comparable to optical colonoscopy

1. Computed tomographic colonography (CTC) and optical colonoscopy (OC) screening strategies resulted in similar detection rates of advanced neoplasia.

2. Rates of positive screening based on polyp size were achieved through CTC with significantly fewer adverse events compared to OC.

Original Date of Publication: October 2007

Study Rundown: Advanced neoplasia of the colon consists of adenocarcinomas and advanced adenomas, the latter of which are associated with a high risk of progression to cancer. Due to their potential to transform into invasive lesions, the early detection and removal of advanced adenomas represent key steps in reducing colorectal cancer mortality. Historically, fecal occult blood testing and sigmoidoscopy were used as primary screening tools. However, it was later found that over a third of colonic polyps are located proximal to the splenic flexure, rendering these methods inadequate in screening the entire colon. It was not until years later that single contrast barium enema (SCBE), and then double contrast barium enema (DCBE) emerged as the first radiologic imaging tests allowing for the detection of colonic neoplasms. Owing to the technically demanding and time-consuming nature of these imaging studies, the barium enema was later replaced by CTC as the primary imaging test used in colorectal cancer screening. In a prior prospective cohort conducted by Yee and colleagues, in which 300 patients underwent CTC followed by standard colonoscopy, CTC had a high sensitivity in the detection of clinically important polyps.

In the present study conducted by Kim and colleagues, CTC was compared to OC in the detection of advanced adenomas and adenocarcinomas. The results of this study showed that the total number of advanced neoplasms detected through CTC was similar to that detected by primary OC, with CTC requiring significantly fewer polypectomies to achieve these outcomes. While the rate of colonic perforations in the primary OC group was within an expected range, no serious complications were reported as a result of CTC.

In-Depth [non-randomized trial]: The results of a CTC screening program were compared to those of an OC screening program. Patients in each study group were consecutively enrolled, with partially overlapping time periods, from the same general screening population and geographic region. Key exclusion criteria included polyp surveillance, history of a bowel disorder (i.e., inflammatory bowel disease), polyposis syndromes, and hereditary nonpolyposis colorectal cancer (HNPCC) syndrome. Polyps were defined as large if measuring at least 10 mm in size, small if between 6-9 mm, and diminutive if 5 mm or less. As part of CTC preparation, 250 mL of 2% barium and 60 mL of diatrizoate were administered to tag residual stool and fluid, respectively. Colon distention was achieved through automated delivery of carbon dioxide. All CTC imaging studies were reviewed by 1 of 5 gastrointestinal radiologists and, where present, polyps were measured with electronic calipers. For all polyps >6 mm, same-day therapeutic OC was offered unless contraindicated. Patients with only 1-2 polyps measuring between 6-9 mm were also given the option of CTC surveillance only. Polyps identified through OC were measured through in vivo OC estimation and removed with standard techniques.

A total of 3120 (mean age 57 years, SD 7.2 years; 44% male) and 3163 patients (mean age 58.1 years, SD 7.8. years; 44% male) underwent primary CTC and primary OC, respectively. Following primary CTC, 246 patients (7.9%) were referred for therapeutic OC. The total number of polyps removed in patients that underwent primary OC was 2434, far exceeding the 561 that were removed in patients who underwent primary CTC ($p < 0.001$). However, there were no statistically significant differences between groups with respect to the number of large ($p = 0.92$) or small ($p = 0.14$) advanced adenomas removed. The two screening strategies also had similar rates of positive screening results based on size threshold for polyps measuring ≥10 mm ($p = 0.06$) and ≥ 6 mm ($p = 0.59$). While there were no perforations or serious complications related to CTC or subsequent therapeutic OC, colonic perforation occurred in 7 (0.2%) patients in the primary OC screening group, of which 4 required surgical repair.

Kim DH, Pickhardt PJ, Taylor AJ, Leung WK, Winter TC, Hinshaw JL, et al. CT colonography versus colonoscopy for the detection of advanced neoplasia. The New England Journal of Medicine. 2007 Oct;357(14):1403-12.

Additional Review:

Levine MS, Yee J. History, Evolution, and Current Status of Radiologic Imaging Tests for Colorectal Cancer Screening. Radiology. 2014 Nov;273(2S):S160-S80.

Yee J, Akerkar GA, Hung RK, Steinauer-Gebauer AM, Wall SD, McQuaid KR. Colorectal Neoplasia: Performance Characteristics of CT Colonography for Detection in 300 Patients 1. Radiology. 2001 Jun;219(3):685-92.

Endovaginal ultrasound highly sensitive screen for endometrial cancer

1. Endovaginal ultrasound (EVUS) revealing an endometrial stripe of 5 mm or greater was 96% sensitive for endometrial cancer and 92% sensitive for other endometrial disease, allowing for noninvasive screening and subsequent determination of candidacy for endometrial biopsy.

2. EVUS was less specific among postmenopausal women utilizing hormone replacement therapy (HRT) than among those who refrained from HRT, and this overall low sensitivity necessitated endometrial biopsy in all women with an abnormal EVUS.

Original Date of Publication: November 1998

Study Rundown: Endometrial cancer is the third most common cancer of the female reproductive tract after ovarian and cervical cancers, but has a low mortality rate if brought to early medical attention. It typically presents with painless, abnormal uterine bleeding among postmenopausal women, particularly those who are obese or utilizing HRT without progesterone supplementation, as unopposed estrogens promote endometrial hyperplasia. Prior to the widespread use of EVUS in screening symptomatic women for endometrial abnormalities, endometrial biopsy was the only diagnostic tool used in the workup of at-risk women with abnormal uterine bleeding. However, endometrial biopsy is invasive, painful, and can be nondiagnostic or inaccurate in over a quarter of attempts. The referenced study reviewed the literature from 1966 to 1996 regarding the use of EVUS as the first-line screening tool among women with suspicion of endometrial cancer in an effort to determine if a negative screening EVUS could obviate the need for endometrial biopsy. Utilizing an endometrial thickness threshold of 5 mm for positivity on any given EVUS examination, the authors found a pooled sensitivity of 96% for the detection of endometrial cancer and 92% for other endometrial disease, including atypical endometrial hyperplasia or endometrial polyps. Additionally, no significant sensitivity difference was found between women using HRT and those not. However, specificity for the detection of endometrial cancer varied significantly between women who did and did not use HRT, finding almost three times as many women on HRT to have an abnormal EVUS despite normal histology on biopsy. Of note, this analysis did not include studies involving women using tamoxifen, which may markedly thicken the endometrium, and also did not evaluate the use of EVUS as a screening tool in asymptomatic women due to the rarity of endometrial cancer. The variability and overall low-to-moderate specificity of EVUS demonstrated it to be an improper tool for the ultimate diagnosis of an endometrial abnormality, but it displayed excellent sensitivity characteristics in the initial workup of at-risk women presenting with abnormal uterine bleeding concerning for malignancy. A negative EVUS result was shown to reduce the pretest odds of cancer by roughly 90% regardless of HRT status, therefore effectively ruling out cancer and preventing unnecessary invasive biopsies.

In-Depth [systematic review and meta-analysis]: This systematic review and meta-analysis pooled data from 35 studies published between 1966 and 1996 examining the use of EVUS in the diagnostic workup of primarily postmenopausal patients with suspected endometrial cancer, all of which were confirmed by endometrial biopsy. A total of 5892 women (mean age 61 years; 471 women using HRT) were included, with 94% presenting with vaginal bleeding. The sensitivity, specificity, and positive and negative predictive values were calculated for EVUS in the detection of both endometrial cancer and other endometrial abnormalities (polyps or atypical hyperplasia), and among women who were and were not utilizing postmenopausal HRT. Within the sampled group, the prevalence of endometrial cancer was calculated to be 13%, while that of endometrial polyps or hyperplasia was 40%. Women with normal endometrial histology displayed a mean endometrial thickness of 4±1 mm, while women with endometrial polyps, hyperplasia and cancer displayed mean thicknesses of 10±3 mm, 14±4 mm and 20±6 mm, respectively. A 5 mm threshold for EVUS positivity was selected as it displayed the best overall sensitivity and specificity characteristics. Regardless of HRT status, the sensitivity of EVUS in testing for endometrial cancer was 96% (95%CI 94-98%), while it was 92% (95%CI 90-93%) in testing for other endometrial abnormalities. This lack of variation despite HRT status and high sensitivity demonstrated that EVUS is highly accurate in the exclusion of endometrial disease, with a negative likelihood ratio of 0.05-0.12. Therefore, in a woman with a 10% pretest probability of endometrial disease, typical for that of postmenopausal women presenting with abnormal uterine bleeding, a negative EVUS reduced her risk of disease to 1%. Regarding specificity, the study found that EVUS cannot accurately distinguish between endometrial cancers, polyps or hyperplasia, necessitating a subsequent endometrial biopsy in all women with an abnormal EVUS. This study definitively established EVUS as an effective first-line tool in the diagnostic workup of women with suspected endometrial cancer while providing the baseline, evidence-based threshold for examination positivity used in current practice.

Smith-Bindman R, Kerlikowske K, Feldstein V, Subak L, Scheidler J, Segal M, Brand R, Grady D. Endovaginal ultrasound to exclude endometrial cancer and other endometrial abnormalities. Journal of the American Medical Association. 1998 Nov 4;280(17):1510–17.

The PLCO trial I: PSA and digital rectal examination in prostate cancer screening

The Prostate, Lung, Colorectal, and Ovarian (PLCO) Cancer Screening Trial is a large population-based randomized trial sponsored by the National Cancer Institute (NCI) to explore the effects of screening on cancer mortality. The trial has been conducted at 10 different centers across the U.S. Participants randomized to the intervention group receive active screening for PLCO cancers (i.e., chest x-ray, flexible sigmoidoscopy, CA-125, transvaginal ultrasound, PSA, digital rectal examination) in the first 6 years of the trial and are subsequently followed for another 7 years. Participants randomized to the usual care group are managed with usual medical care and are followed for 13 years. The trial began in 1993 and the screening phase of the trial was completed in 2006. We report below on the findings regarding prostate cancer screening using PSA testing and digital rectal examination.

1. Subjects who underwent annual prostate-specific antigen (PSA) testing for 6 years and annual digital rectal examination (DRE) for 4 years had a significantly increased incidence of prostate cancer compared to usual care.

2. Screening with PSA testing and DRE did not significantly reduce mortality from prostate cancer compared to usual care.

Original Date of Publication: March 2009

Study Rundown: The combination of PSA testing and DRE was the standard screening approach for prostate cancer for several decades. While many clinicians used this approach, there was significant uncertainty regarding the benefits and harms of prostate cancer screening. This led to the release of conflicting guidelines from different organizations, such as the American Cancer Society and the U.S. Preventative Task Force (USPSTF). The prostate component of the PLCO trial assessed the effect of annual PSA testing for 6 years and annual DRE for 4 years on mortality rates from prostate cancer. The study revealed that screening with PSA testing and DRE was associated with an increased incidence of prostate cancer, but not with a significant reduction in mortality when compared with usual care. Thus, the concern was that prostate cancer screening may expose patients to the risks of overdiagnosis and overtreatment of prostate cancer, with no actual benefit in survival.

The limitations of this study included a relatively high PSA testing and DRE rate in the control group, ranging from 40%-52% for PSA testing and 41%-46% for DRE. This rate of screening in the control group may have reduced the relative difference in prostate cancer mortality between the control and screening groups. Secondly, about 44% of subjects in both groups had undergone 1 or more PSA tests at baseline, which may have excluded more easily detectable cancers prior to the enrollment in the study, thereby also potentially leading to a reduction in the observed difference in prostate cancer mortality. Finally, it is possible that improvements in prostate cancer therapy equally reduced death from prostate cancer in both experimental groups, thereby dampening the survival benefits of early cancer detection from screening. In summary, the prostate component of the PLCO trial found that screening with PSA testing and DRE was not associated with significant decreases in prostate cancer mortality.

In-Depth [randomized controlled trial]: The PLCO trial was a randomized, controlled trial that enrolled 154 900 participants between 55-74 years of age from 10 study centers in the U.S. The exclusion criteria were a history of PLCO cancer, current cancer treatment, and more than one instance of PSA testing in the 3 years prior to enrollment. Of the enrolled participants, 38 343 were assigned to the screening group that received annual PSA testing for 6 years and annual DRE for 4 years, while 38 350 were assigned to the control group. Follow-up remains planned for all subjects for at least 13 years, but the results of this study were released with at least 7 years of follow-up for all patients and 10 years of follow-up for 67% of the patients due to public health considerations raised by the study's results. At 7 years, more subjects in the screening group were diagnosed with prostate cancer than in the control group (rate ratio 1.22; 95%CI 1.16-1.29). This difference persisted for patients with 10 years of follow-up (rate ratio 1.17; 95%CI 1.11-1.22). There was, however, no significant difference in mortality from prostate cancer between the screening and control groups at 7 years (rate ratio 1.16; 95%CI 0.76-1.76) or 10 years of follow-up (rate ratio 1.09; 95%CI 0.76-1.76).

Andriole GL, Crawford ED, Grubb RL, Buys SS, Chia D, Church TR, et al. Mortality Results from a Randomized Prostate-Cancer Screening Trial. The New England Journal of Medicine. 2009 Mar 26;360(13):1310–9.

The PLCO trial II: Ovarian cancer screening does not reduce mortality

1. Randomization of patients to either yearly ovarian cancer screening with transvaginal ultrasound (TVUS) and serum CA-125 levels or usual care did not significantly reduce cancer-related mortality.

2. False-positive results among the screening cohort were associated with significant surgical morbidity, with at least one serious complication suffered by roughly one-sixth of those who underwent surgical workup.

Original Date of Publication: June 2011

Study Rundown: Ovarian cancer remains both a diagnostic and therapeutic dilemma: it is often diagnosed late in its course due to vague and nonspecific presenting symptoms, and has poor long-term survival rates once it has spread beyond a single ovary. However, surgically managed ovarian cancers that remain confined to the ovary display 5-year survival rates greater than 90%, suggesting that early recognition and treatment could lead to a substantial mortality benefit. The referenced trial, part of a series of the PLCO, randomized women to either yearly screening for ovarian cancer with TVUS for 3 years and measurement of serum CA-125 levels for 5 years, or standard care with yearly bimanual examination in an effort to determine if ovarian cancer screening would yield earlier diagnoses and resultant prognostic improvements. Screening did not significantly increase the number of cases of ovarian cancer diagnosed, though the results did trend toward significance. More poignantly however, the distributions of cancer stage at diagnosis were similar between groups, with a majority diagnosed at stage III-IV, and therefore ovarian cancer-related survival remained similarly low between groups. Screening was itself not a benign intervention, with positive findings frequently requiring surgical management. Nearly 10% of women in the screening cohort had false-positive results, requiring the performance of ultimately unnecessary surgeries in which 15% of patients suffered at least one serious post-surgical complication. This trial demonstrated that annual screening with simultaneous TVUS and CA-125 does not reduce cancer-specific mortality among average risk women, but does increase the risk of harm related to the performance of invasive procedures, particularly when due to false-positive findings or overdiagnosis.

In-Depth [randomized controlled trial]: A total of 68 557 women (roughly 88.5% of non-Hispanic white ethnicity, primarily aged 55-64 years) of average risk for ovarian cancer were enrolled at 10 screening centers across the United States. Subjects were excluded from analysis if they had a pretrial history of ovarian cancer or bilateral oophorectomy. Women were randomized to either the screening arm of the trial, in which they underwent yearly TVUS for 3 years, and yearly serum CA-125 measurements for 4-6 years, or the control arm of the trial, in which they underwent only yearly bimanual examination. Due to the invasive nature of the screening tests, no blinding could be performed. The positivity threshold for TVUS included ovarian volume greater than 10 cm^3, cyst volume greater than 10 cm^3, complex ovarian cysts with solid or papillary projections into the cavity, or any mixed (solid or cystic) components within a cystic ovarian tumor. Of note, this size threshold may have been too high to effectively detect low stage ovarian tumors, which are thought to be less than 10 cm^3, but would have introduced further false-negative results. A positivity threshold of 35 U/mL was used for serum CA-125 levels. A total of 212 cases of ovarian cancer were detected in the screening arm (5.7 per 10 000 person-years) while 176 cases were detected in the control group (4.7 per 10 000 person-years; RR 1.21; 95%CI 0.99-1.48) during the mean 12.6 year follow-up period. Of the cancers detected, the majority were high grade serous cystadenocarcinomas in both groups with a similar distribution of histological subtypes and grades. No stage shift, or difference in the cancer stage at time of diagnosis, was observed between groups. The majority of tumors were diagnosed at stage III-IV, with 69% of those detected during screening being advanced stage, as compared to 78% in the control group. As a stage shift is believed to be necessary for a mortality benefit, no significant difference in cancer-related mortality was noted between the two groups (RR, 1.18; 95%CI 0.82-1.71). A total of 3285 (9.6%) women suffered false-positive screening results, 1080 of whom underwent surgical management as part of their diagnostic workup. Of these women, 163 (15%) suffered at least one major surgical complication. This trial demonstrated that screening for ovarian cancer with TVUS and serum CA-125 levels does not reduce cancer stage at the time of diagnosis or cancer-related mortality, and may in fact introduce potential harm related to the workup of false-positive results.

Buys SS, Partridge E, Black A, Johnson CC, Lamerato L, Isaacs C, et al. Effect of screening on ovarian cancer mortality: The prostate, lung, colorectal and ovarian (PLCO) cancer screening randomized controlled trial. Journal of the American Medical Association. 2011 Jun 8;305(22):2295–303.

The PLCO trial III: Flexible sigmoidoscopy in colon cancer screening

1. Compared to usual care, screening with flexible sigmoidoscopy significantly reduced the incidence of colon cancer in the distal and proximal colon.

2. Screening with flexible sigmoidoscopy significantly reduced mortality cancers of the distal colon only when compared with usual care.

Original Date of Publication: June 2012

Study Rundown: Colon cancer screening with fecal occult blood testing (FOBT) was previously reported to reduce colon cancer incidence and mortality. Flexible sigmoidoscopy is an endoscopic procedure where the most distal segment of the colon is examined. Previous studies conducted in Europe suggested that sigmoidoscopy was associated with reductions in both colon cancer incidence and mortality. The colorectal component of the PLCO trial assessed the effect of screening with two flexible sigmoidoscopies, spaced 3 or 5 years apart, on the incidence of and mortality from colon cancer in patients from the U.S. This study demonstrated that screening with flexible sigmoidoscopy was associated with a significant reduction in incidence of both distal and proximal colon cancer, regardless of the stage of the cancer, when compared to the usual-care group. Screening was also associated with a significant reduction in mortality independent of cancer stage, but only for distal colon cancer. For proximal colon cancer, screening resulted in reduced mortality for cancers staged I, II, or III, but not IV.

Study limitations included a substantial rate of endoscopy use in the usual-care group during the time the intervention group was undergoing screening - 46.5% of the usual-care group underwent either a flexible sigmoidoscopy or colonoscopy. This use may have dampened the difference in incidence and mortality between the usual-care and screening groups. In summary, the colorectal component of the PLCO trial found that screening with flexible sigmoidoscopy was associated with decreased colon cancer mortality and incidence. The study results support routine screening with flexible sigmoidoscopy followed by colonoscopy for cases of abnormal screening results.

In-Depth [randomized controlled trial]: The PLCO cancer trial was a randomized, controlled trial that enrolled 154 900 participants between 55-74 years of age from 10 study centers in the U.S. The primary exclusion criteria were a history of PLCO cancer, ongoing cancer treatment, and lower endoscopy (i.e., flexible sigmoidoscopy, colonoscopy, or barium enema) in the previous 3 years. Of the enrolled participants, 77 445 were randomized to receive flexible sigmoidoscopy at baseline and again after 3 or 5 years, while the other 77 455 were assigned to receive usual care. The primary endpoint was death from colon cancer, while secondary endpoints included colorectal cancer incidence, cancer stage, survival, harms of screening, and all-cause mortality. The primary analysis was an intention-to-screen comparison of mortality between the two experimental groups.

At a median follow-up of 11.9 years, the intervention group experienced a significant 21% reduction in colon cancer incidence compared to the usual care group (RR 0.79; 95%CI 0.72-0.85). This reduction was observed for both distal colon cancer (RR 0.71, 95%CI 0.64-0.80) and proximal colon cancer (RR 0.86; 95%CI 0.76-0.97). Additionally, there was a 26% reduction in colon cancer mortality due to screening (RR 0.74; 95%CI 0.63-0.87). This reduction was only significant for distal colon cancer (RR 0.50; 95%CI 0.38-0.64), but not proximal colon cancer (RR 0.97; 95%CI 0.77-1.22).

Schoen RE, Pinsky PF, Weissfeld JL, Yokochi LA, Church T, Laiyemo AO, et al. Colorectal-Cancer Incidence and Mortality with Screening Flexible Sigmoidoscopy. New England Journal of Medicine. 2012 Jun 21;366(25):2345–57.

PI-RADS version 2: Standardized acquisition, interpretation, and reporting of prostate MRI

1. A joint steering committee have revised the original Prostate Imaging Reporting and Data System (PI-RADS) guidelines to form PI-RADS version 2 (v2), which improves the standardization of imaging acquisition and reporting in pre-therapy patients with suspected prostate cancer.

2. DWI is the predominant sequence to evaluate peripheral zone (PZ) lesions, while T2-weighted magnetic resonance imaging (MRI) is favored for evaluation of the transition zone (TZ).

3. Lesions with a PI-RADS score of ≥3 should be reported. If multiple, up to 4 should be reported with the index lesion identified.

4. The guidelines are intended to evolve as the prostate imaging community gains clinical experience in the application of PI-RADS v2.

Original Date of Publication: April 2015

Study Rundown: The European Society of Urogenital Radiology (ESUR) originally published the Prostate Imaging Reporting and Data System (PI-RADS) in 2012 to provide structured clinical guidelines for multiparametric prostate magnetic resonance imaging (mpMRI) using evidenced-based data and consensus expert opinion. This guideline was updated in 2015 by a steering committee formed by the American College of Radiology (ACR), ESUR, and AdMeTech Foundation to standardize and reduce the inter-center variability in imaging acquisition and reporting, and to improve characterization and risk stratification of patients undergoing imaging for suspected prostate cancer.

In the original version, prostatic abnormalities were scored based on individual pulse sequences on mpMRI; including T2-weighted, diffusion weighted imaging and apparent diffusion coefficient (DWI-ADC), dynamic contrast-enhanced (DCE) imaging, and (optionally) MR spectroscopy. Although the guidelines carried information regarding risk stratification, enrollment criteria for active surveillance programs, and recommendations for imaging protocols, it failed to specify how the individual sequences contributed to an overall score. This resulted in between-center variability in image acquisition and reporting.

Compared to the original version, PI-RADS v2 is more precise in its scope and purpose. It includes an overview of normal prostate anatomy, benign findings, terminology, and provides specific recommendations to assign an overall score. The following are several key differences between the original and PI-RADS v2:

- The guidelines are explicit that they only apply to pre-therapy patients being evaluated for prostate cancer, not for follow-up or post-treatment assessment.
- Only minimal technical parameters for acceptable mpMRI are given.
- MR spectroscopy is omitted and DCE is assigned a minor role.
- The overall score is based only on mpMRI, without contribution from clinical factors.

PI-RADS v2 has also defined the predominant sequence for evaluation, based on the zonal location of the abnormality; DWI for PZ lesions and T2-weighted MRI for TZ lesions. Other sequences are considered ancillary for equivocal lesions. DCE is no longer evaluated on a 5-point scale and is now either positive or negative. The 5-point scale used to evaluate DWI-ADC and T2-weighted MRI are retained from the original version. The score based on the predominant sequence is used for an overall score assignment and interpretation of cancer risk:

PI-RADS 1 – Very low (clinically significant cancer is highly unlikely to be present)

PI-RADS 2 – Low (clinically significant cancer is unlikely to be present)

PI-RADS 3 - Intermediate (the presence of clinically significant cancer is equivocal)

PI-RADS 4 – High (clinically significant cancer is likely to be present)

PI-RADS 5 - Very high (clinically significant cancer is highly likely to be present)

The following is the scoring classification for PZ and TZ lesions based on the appearance on ADC and high-*b* value DWI, PZ lesions based on T2-weighted MRI, and TZ lesions based on T2-weighted MRI, respectively. Please see Tables I and II for further detail:

PZ or TZ lesions based on DWI-ADC:

1. Normal on ADC maps or high-*b* value DWI
2. Indistinct hypointense abnormality on ADC
3. Focal mild to moderate hypointense abnormality on ADC and isointense to mild hyperintense on high-*b* value DWI
4. Focal markedly hypointense abnormality on ADC and markedly hyperintense on high-*b* value DWI; ≤1.5 cm in greatest dimension
5. Same as 4), but ≥1.5 cm in greatest dimension or definite extraprostatic extension

PZ abnormalities based on T2-weighted MRI:

1. Uniformly hyperintense (normal)
2. Linear, wedge-shaped, or diffuse mild hypointensity, usually indistinct margin
3. Noncircumscribed, rounded, moderate hypointensity
4. Circumscribed, homogenous moderately hypointense focus or mass confined to the prostate; ≤1.5 cm in greatest dimension
5. Same as 4), but ≥1.5 cm in greatest dimension or definite extraprostatic extension

TZ abnormalities based on T2-weighted MRI:

1. Homogenous intermediate signal intensity (normal)
2. Circumscribed hypointense or heterogenous encapsulated nodule(s)
3. Heterogenous signal intensity with obscured margins
4. Noncircumscribed, homogenous moderately hypointense focus or mass confined to the prostate; ≤1.5 cm in greatest dimension
5. Same as 4), but ≥1.5 cm in greatest dimension or definite extraprostatic extension

A maximum of 4 lesions with an overall score of 3, 4, or 5 are reported, with the index lesion identified. A PI-RADS score is reported for each lesion. A standardized format for reporting is recommended, though no specific model is given. The guidelines are intended to evolve with time, as radiologists gain experience in the clinical application of the PI-RADS v2 system.

ACR. PI-RADS - American College of Radiology [Internet]. 2015 [cited 2017 May 14]. Available from: https://www.acr.org/Quality-Safety/Resources/PIRADS

Additional Review:

Hamoen EHJ, de Rooij M, Witjes JA, Barentsz JO, Rovers MM. Use of the Prostate Imaging Reporting and Data System (PI-RADS) for Prostate Cancer Detection with Multiparametric Magnetic Resonance Imaging: A Diagnostic Meta-analysis. Eur Urol. 2015 Jun;67(6):1112–21.

PI-RADS Framework – Transition Zone Lesions			
T2W	DWI	DCE	PI-RADS
1	Any*	Any	1
2	Any	Any	2
3	≤4	Any	3
	5	Any	4
4	Any	Any	4
5	Any	Any	5

Table I. PI-RADS v2 scoring system for transition zone lesions. *Any indicates 1-5. Table compiled with information from https://www.acr.org/Quality-Safety/Resources/BIRADS.

PI-RADS Framework – Peripheral Zone Lesions			
DWI	T2W	DCE	PI-RADS
1	Any*	Any	1
2	Any	Any	2
3	Any	-	3
		+	4
4	Any	Any	4
5	Any	Any	5

Table II. PI-RADS v2 scoring system for peripheral zone lesions. *Any indicates 1-5. Table compiled with information from https://www.acr.org/Quality-Safety/Resources/BIRADS.

Kocher Criteria differentiates pediatric septic arthritis and transient synovitis of the hip

1. Children with septic arthritis of the hip could be accurately differentiated from transient synovitis of the hip on the basis of the presence or absence of four major clinical predictors: fever, lack of weight-bearing status, erythrocyte sedimentation rate (ESR) >40 mm/hr, and leukocytosis greater than 12 000 cells/cm^3.

2. Several other variables increased the odds of septic arthritis, including radiographic evidence of joint effusion, fever with chills, female gender, and recent antibiotic use.

Original Date of Publication: December 1999

Study Rundown: When evaluating a child with acute hip pain, only a few diagnoses can be made primarily by radiographic appearance, including Legg-Calve-Perthes disease, slipped capital femoral epiphysis, and fracture. Differentiating between septic arthritis and transient synovitis of the hip remains a diagnostic dilemma. The appropriate management of septic arthritis requires timely initiation of intravenous antibiotics and surgical drainage of the infected joint, thus making rapid and accurate diagnosis vital in avoiding both the sequelae of a failure to treat and of the morbidity associated with treatment of those without a septic joint.

In the reviewed article, Kocher et al. set out to simplify the diagnostic process in differentiating between a septic hip and transient synovitis by developing and validating a set of clinical criteria by which an individual's risk for septic arthritis may be stratified. In a retrospective review of all cases of an acutely irritable hip in children between 1979 and 1996 at a major pediatric tertiary-care hospital, several variables were found to significantly differ between those with true septic arthritis and those with transient synovitis of the hip. The four variables that were most predictive of true septic arthritis were a history of fever, an inability to bear weight on the affected hip, an ESR greater than 40 mm/hr, and a leukocytosis of greater than 12 000 cells/cm^3. Patients with all four criteria were 99.6% likely to have septic arthritis, while those with zero of four criteria had septic arthritis effectively ruled out with less than 0.2% probability of an infected joint. Patients with true septic arthritis were also significantly more likely to be female, present with chills, have recent antibiotic use, and demonstrate radiographic evidence of a joint effusion at the affected site, although these features were not included in the final clinical decision algorithm due to reduced specificity. Following publication, Caird et al. prospectively evaluated these criteria in a separate pediatric population, finding that the algorithm remained effective, but inclusion of a C-reactive protein >2.0 mg/dL was additionally predictive of septic arthritis as a fifth criterion and was independently more valuable than an ESR. However, with further prospective use of the Kocher criteria in alternative pediatric populations, such as that published in Luhmann et al. and rebutted by Kocher et al. in 2004, the clinical prediction rules demonstrated reduced but still reasonable diagnostic performance, possibly due to suboptimal modeling of the selected variables within a new population. This algorithm was the first and remains a lasting and effective evidence-based guideline for the clinical differentiation of septic arthritis from transient synovitis of the hip across multiple pediatric populations.

In-Depth [retrospective cohort]: A total of 282 children presenting with acute irritability of the hip between 1979 and 1996 at a major Northeastern pediatric hospital were included in this retrospective review. Patients were excluded if they presented with complicating factors, including immunocompromised status, renal failure, neonatal sepsis, postoperative hip infection, juvenile rheumatoid arthritis, subsequent development of Legg-Calve-Perthes disease or associated proximal femoral osteomyelitis. Patients were stratified into one of three categories of disease: True septic arthritis (38 patients), proven by positive bacterial growth from synovial fluid aspirate with associated fluid white blood cell (WBC) count >50 000 cells/cm^3; presumed septic arthritis (44 patients) on the basis of a synovial fluid aspirate with > 50 000 WBCs/cm^3 but no bacterial growth on culture; or transient synovitis of the hip (86 patients), with <50 000 WBCs/cm^3 on synovial aspiration, no bacterial growth on culture, and spontaneous resolution of symptoms without antibiotics or surgery. Multiple clinical variables were tracked to determine which differed most significantly between groups by univariate analysis and multiple logistic regression analysis.

Overall, children with true septic arthritis were significantly more likely to be female, and present with a history positive for fever >38.5 degrees Celsius, chills, recent antibiotic use, radiographic evidence of a joint effusion, non-weight bearing status on the affected side, elevated ESR, reduced hematocrit, and leukocytosis ($p < 0.05$ for all). On further analysis, the four variables that were most predictive of septic arthritis formed the final Kocher Criteria and included fever >38.5C, non-weight bearing status, ESR >40 mm/hr, and leukocytosis >12 000 WBC/cm^3. Meeting zero of the four criteria effectively ruled out septic arthritis (probability <0.2%), while meeting all four criteria effectively ruled it in (probability of 99.6%). With three of four criteria met, probability of disease was 93.1%, which reduced to 40.0% for two criteria and 3% for one criteria.

Kocher MS, Zurakowski D, Kasser JR. Differentiating between septic arthritis and transient synovitis of the hip in children: An evidence-based clinical prediction algorithm. The Journal of Bone and Joint Surgery. 1999 Dec 1;81-A(12):1662–70.

Additional Review:

Kocher MS, Mandiga R, Murphy JM, Goldmann D, Harper M, Sundel R, et al. A clinical practice guideline for treatment of septic arthritis in children: Efficacy in improving process of care and effect on outcome of septic arthritis of the hip. The Journal of Bone and Joint Surgery. 2003 June 1;85-A(6):994–99.

Caird MS, Flynn JM, Leung YL, Millman JE, D'Italia JG, Dormans JP. Factors distinguishing septic arthritis from transient synovitis of the hip in children: a prospective study. The Journal of Bone and Joint Surgery. 2006 June 1;88-A(6):1251–57.

Luhmann SJ, Jones A, Schootman M, Gordon JE, Schoenecker PL, Luhmann JD. Differentiation between septic arthritis and transient synovitis of the hip in children with clinical prediction algorithms. The Journal of Bone and Joint Surgery. 2004 May 1;86-A(5):956–62.

Kocher Criteria
1. Non weight-bearing 2. Temp >38.5 C/101.3 F 3. ESR >40 mm/hr 4. WBC >12 000 cells/mm^2

Table I. Kocher criteria.

III. Interventional Literature

"Science is built up of facts, as a house is built of stones; but an accumulation of facts is no more a science than a heap of stones is a house."

- Henri Poincaré, PhD

The RAPTURE trial: Radiofrequency ablation effective and safe in lung cancer

1. Percutaneous radiofrequency ablation (RFA) demonstrated robust levels of efficacy and safety in patients with malignant lung cancers who were poor candidates for surgery.

2. RFA was only performed in lung tumors less than 3.5 cm in diameter in this cohort.

Original Date of Publication: July 2008

Study Rundown: Primary lung cancer is the leading cause of death in the United States with over 160 000 deaths annually. Lungs are also a frequent site of metastasis from colorectal, breast, and renal cancers. Traditional treatment of malignant lung cancers primarily involved surgical resection. However, this excluded a large group of patients with reduced pulmonary reserve or comorbid conditions who were deemed poor surgical candidates. A previous retrospective review by Simon et al. demonstrated in a cohort of 153 patients that CT-guided RFA of lung tumors were associated with robust rates of safety and promising long-term survival rates. The purpose of this landmark prospective trial was to determine the safety and efficacy of RFA in malignant lung cancers.

The trial prospectively followed over 100 patients with either non-small cell lung cancer (NSCLC) or lung metastasis that was deemed ineligible for other curative treatments. The trial only included patients with up to three tumors per lung with no tumor larger than 3.5 cm in diameter. The primary outcome was technical success, safety, and confirmed response as determined by a 1-month follow-up CT scan. At the conclusion of the trial, technical success was achieved in 99% of patients with no significant changes to pulmonary function or procedure-related deaths within the study group. Complete clinical response was maintained in 88% of patients at 1-year post procedure, with no difference in responsiveness between tumor subtypes. The study is limited by the relatively small sample size and the lack of efficacy data for masses greater than 3.5 cm due to the technical size limitations of the ablation sphere. Additionally, Simons et al. and others have shown poorer clinical outcome for patients with tumor greater than 3 cm in size. Given the lack of current randomized controlled trials in this population, this was one of the first trials to demonstrate prospectively the robust technical feasibility and safety profile of RFA in the treatment of malignant lung cancers.

In-Depth [prospective cohort]: This study was a prospective, intention-to-treat, multi-center clinical trial of 106 patients from seven centers in Europe, United States, and Australia. Patients with pathology-proven NSCLC (n=33), or metastasis from other primary cancers (n=73) were included. All patients were deemed a non-surgical candidate or unfit for additional radiotherapy or chemotherapy. Key exclusion criteria included patients with greater than three tumors per lung, tumor size of 3.5 cm or greater, or patients with previous pneumonectomy. RFA was performed by a 150-200 W generators with a deployment device with a maximum ablation sphere of 5 cm in diameter. Post-procedure, patients were schedule for follow-up at 3 months intervals for up to two years. The primary outcome of interest was the technical success, safety, and rate of confirmed clinical response. Clinical response was defined as a reduction in tumor size of at least 30% with no evidence of tumor growth or contrast enhancement on follow-up CT scan. Secondary outcomes were overall and cancer-specific survival. At the conclusion of the trial, technical success was achieved in 105 of 106 (99%) patients. With respect to complications, 20% of patients experienced symptomatic pneumothorax requiring chest tube drainage, however, there were no procedural-related deaths or worsening of pulmonary function performance post-RFA. Confirmed clinical response of treated lesions was demonstrated in 88% of the patient cohort. There were no differences noted in tumor response between cancer subtypes. Overall, the two-year cancer-specific survival rate for patients with NSCLC, colorectal metastases, and other primary metastases were 73% (95%CI 0.54 to 0.86), 68% (95%CI 0.54 to 0.80), and 67% (95%CI 0.48 to 0.84), respectively.

Lencioni R, Crocetti L, Cioni R, Suh R, Glenn D, Regge D, et al. Response to radiofrequency ablation of pulmonary tumors: a prospective, intention-to-treat, multicentre clinical trial (the RAPTURE study). Lancet Oncol. 2008 Jul;9(7):621–8.

Additional Review:

Simon CJ, Dupuy DE, DiPetrillo TA, Safran HP, Grieco CA, Ng T, et al. Pulmonary Radiofrequency Ablation: Long-term Safety and Efficacy in 153 Patients. Radiology. 2007 Apr 1;243(1):268–75.

The ISAT: Endovascular coiling superior to neurosurgical clipping in selected patients with aneurysmal subarachnoid hemorrhage

1. In patients with aneurysmal subarachnoid hemorrhage (SAH), endovascular coiling demonstrated significantly improved survival compared to neurosurgical clipping.

2. Patients with ruptured posterior and middle cerebral arteries were underrepresented in the cohort due to expert consensus for preferential endovascular coiling and neurosurgical clipping, respectively.

Original Date of Publication: October 2002

Study Rundown: Ruptured intracranial aneurysms are the most common cause of spontaneous SAH and are associated with significant morbidity and mortality. Historically, management options have included open neurosurgical clipping and endovascular therapy with detachable coiling. Choice of treatment was previously based on a combination of clinical judgement and the availability of technical expertise in endovascular therapy at referral centers. The purpose of the landmark International Subarachnoid Aneurysm Trial (ISAT) was to compare the safety and efficacy of endovascular coiling to neurosurgical clipping in patients deemed suitable for either treatment.

The ISAT trial randomized over 2000 patients with aneurysmal SAH to either neurosurgical clipping or endovascular coiling. At the conclusion of the trial, endovascular coiling demonstrated a 23% relative risk and 7% absolute risk reduction in significant disability or death compared to surgical clipping. The results of the ISAT trial thus favored endovascular clipping over surgical clipping in the treatment of ruptured intracranial aneurysm. However, extrapolation of these findings to all patients and aneurysm types was limited by the narrow scope of the ISAT population. During the enrollment phase of the trial, 80% of patients screened were excluded for not meeting the requirement for their aneurysm to be judged as equally amenable to neurosurgical or endovascular therapy. Over 80% of the included patients had aneurysms in the anterior cerebral or internal carotid artery. Posterior circulation and middle cerebral artery aneurysms were underrepresented due to expert consensus for preferential endovascular coiling and neurosurgical clipping, respectively; thus the results of ISAT were not applicable to these patient populations.

In-Depth [randomized controlled trial]: The ISAT trial was an open-labeled, multicenter randomized controlled trial that compared the efficacy and safety of endovascular coiling to neurosurgical clipping in patients with SAH secondary to a ruptured intracranial aneurysm. Patients were screened in all participating centers if they had imaging-confirmed SAH and intracranial aneurysm. Patients were evaluated by both a neurosurgeon and an interventional radiologist and were included if the target lesion was felt to equally amenable to either endovascular coiling or neurosurgical clipping. The primary end-point was overall disability or survival at 2 months and 1 year, as measured by the modified Rankin scale. Secondary outcomes included rates of hospital admission or episodes of re-bleeding. The trial was stopped after the planned interim analysis at 1 year.

Overall, 2143 patients out of 9559 screened met the inclusion/exclusion criteria and were randomized. There were no significant differences in baseline characteristics between the group randomized to endovascular treatment (n=1073) and neurosurgery (n=1070). However, 83% of patients had aneurysms in the anterior cerebral or internal carotid arteries. Patients with posterior circulation and middle cerebral artery aneurysms represented only 2.7% and 14.1% of patients, respectively. At the conclusion of the trial, patients randomized to endovascular coiling demonstrated significantly lower rates of disability or death at 1 year compared to surgical clipping (23.7% versus 30.6%; $p = 0.019$). Patients in the endovascular group had a relative- and absolute risk reduction of disability or death of 22.6% (95%CI 8.9% to 34.2%) and 6.9% (2.5% to 11.3%), respectively. The risk of re-bleeding after 1-year was 2 per 1276 patients in the endovascular group and 0 per 1081 patients in the neurosurgery group.

Molyneux A. International Subarachnoid Aneurysm Trial (ISAT) of neurosurgical clipping versus endovascular coiling in 2143 patients with ruptured intracranial aneurysms: a randomised trial. The Lancet. 2002 Oct 26;360(9342):1267–74.

The CREST: Stenting versus endarterectomy for carotid stenosis

1. The rate of stroke, myocardial infarction or death did not differ significantly between patients treated with carotid artery stenting (CAS) compared to carotid endarterectomy (CEA).

2. The periprocedural rate of stroke was higher with stenting, while the rate of myocardial infarction was higher with endarterectomy.

Original Date of Publication: July 2010

Study Rundown: Carotid artery stenosis occurs as a result of atherosclerosis and leads to increasing risk of embolus and stroke. CEA and CAS are two procedures used to treat carotid artery stenosis but the evidence regarding their comparative efficacies was inconclusive. The Carotid Revascularization Endarterectomy versus Stenting Trial (CREST) is one of the largest randomized controlled trials comparing these two treatment modalities. Prior to publication of these results, several trials had found higher rates of stroke and death associated with CAS, leading to a trend towards endarterectomy. The CREST trial found no significant difference in a composite outcome of stroke, myocardial infarction, and death between the two treatment groups and achieved lower rates of complications in both groups than those observed in previous trials. This supported both procedures as safe and effective treatment options; however, these results have been attributed to the highly-trained interventionists involved in the study, which limits the external validity of the results. An interesting finding of the trial was that the rate of periprocedural stroke was higher in the stenting group, while the rate of myocardial infarction was higher in the endarterectomy group. This has led to debate regarding the relative harmful effects of suffering a stroke compared to myocardial infarction with some agreement that stroke results in more debilitating long-term consequences. In summary, the results of the CREST trial did not identify a definitive superior treatment for carotid artery stenosis. Treatment decisions should be individualized to patients' characteristics and needs.

In-Depth [randomized controlled trial]: This trial enrolled 2522 patients from 117 centers in the United States and Canada with symptomatic or asymptomatic carotid stenosis and randomized participants to receive CAS or CEA. Patients were considered eligible if they were symptomatic with ≥50% stenosis on angiography, ≥70% stenosis on ultrasonography, or ≥70% stenosis on computed tomographic/magnetic resonance angiography (CTA/MRA) but

50-69% stenosis on ultrasonography. Partway through the study, eligibility criteria were expanded to include asymptomatic patients with ≥60% stenosis on angiography, ≥70% stenosis on ultrasonography, or ≥80% stenosis on CTA/MRA but 50-69% stenosis on ultrasonography. Exclusion criteria included severe prior stroke, chronic atrial fibrillation, or paroxysmal atrial fibrillation. The primary outcome was a composite of stroke, myocardial infarction, and death during the periprocedural period, or ipsilateral stroke within four years of randomization.

There was no significant difference in the 4-year rates of the primary endpoint between CAS and CEA for the sample as a whole (HR 1.11; 95%CI 0.81-1.51), nor among symptomatic or asymptomatic patients separately ($p = 0.84$). The rate of the primary endpoint during the periprocedural period did not differ between treatment groups; however, when components were analyzed separately, the rate of stroke was higher with CAS (4.1% versus 2.3%, $p = 0.01$) while the rate of myocardial infarction was higher with CEA (1.1% versus 2.3%, $p = 0.03$). Treatment effect was not modified by symptomatic status or sex; however, an interaction was detected between age and treatment efficacy, with CAS more effective in younger patients and CEA more effective in older patients.

Brott TG, Hobson RW, Howard G, Roubin GS, Clark WM, Brooks W, et al. Stenting versus Endarterectomy for Treatment of Carotid-Artery Stenosis. New England Journal of Medicine. 2010 Jul 1;363(1):11–23.

2015 Intraarterial therapy and t-PA trials: MR-CLEAN, EXTEND-IA, ESCAPE, SWIFT PRIME, REVASCAT

1. Across several randomized controlled trials (Table I), patients treated with intraarterial therapy and intravenous (IV) tissue plasminogen activator (t-PA) had consistently improved functional outcomes compared to patients that received IV t-PA alone.

2. Patients were more likely to achieve successful reperfusion after receiving both intraarterial and medical therapy.

3. The addition of intraarterial therapy to usual care did not increase rates of mortality or serious adverse events.

Original Dates of Publication: Multiple 2015 Trials

Study Rundowns: The intravenous (IV) administration of alteplase, a tissue plasminogen activator (t-PA) involved in the breakdown of blood clots, has long been the mainstay in treating acute ischemic stroke. However, a narrow therapeutic time window and various contraindications (i.e., recent surgery, coagulation abnormalities, history of intracranial hemorrhage) have limited the number of patients who qualify for t-PA therapy. IV alteplase is also less effective in penetrating through proximal occlusions of major intracranial arteries, which account for over a third of acute anterior circulation strokes. Intraarterial therapy includes the chemical dissolution of clots with locally delivered thrombolytic agents and/or clot retrieval through thrombectomy with mechanical devices. While a number of trials have been conducted to evaluate the efficacy of intraarterial therapy compared to more conventional treatment, concerns surrounding the design and execution of these studies left uncertainty on the role of intraarterial therapy in managing acute ischemic stroke in conjunction with alteplase.

MR CLEAN

As part of the Multicenter Randomized Clinical Trial of Endovascular Treatment for Acute Ischemic Stroke in the Netherlands (MR CLEAN), patients with proximal arterial occlusion in the anterior cerebral circulation received intraarterial treatment with usual care or usual care alone. Berkhemer and colleagues found that at 90 days of follow-up, patients that received intraarterial therapy in addition to usual care had significantly improved functional outcomes. The results of computed tomography angiography (CTA) also showed that after 24 hours, patients assigned to the intervention group were significantly less likely to have residual occlusion. There were no significant differences in the occurrence of serious adverse events; however, a higher proportion of patients from the interventional group demonstrated clinical signs of a new ischemic stroke in a different vascular territory. Given the invasive nature of intraarterial therapy, these patients were also subject to procedure-related complications not seen in the control group.

EXTEND-IA

Campbell and colleagues subsequently conducted the Emergency Neurological Deficits – Intraarterial (EXTEND-IA) trial to evaluate whether the use of computed tomographic (CT) perfusion imaging could be used in maximizing the therapeutic potential of intraarterial interventions. Specifically, CT perfusion imaging was used to identify patients with a dual target of vessel occlusion and evidence of salvageable tissue; patients with large ischemic cores and without evidence of clinically significant salvageable ischemic brain tissue were not included in the study. Unlike the MR CLEAN trial where various forms of intraarterial therapy were employed, patients in this study received intraarterial therapy using a stent retriever and IV alteplase, or alteplase alone within 6 hours of stroke onset. As the results of an interim analysis strongly favored the intervention, this trial was stopped early, demonstrating that CT perfusion imaging can be effectively used to identify patients with the greatest potential to benefit from endovascular therapy. Specifically, early combination endovascular therapy and IV alteplase was associated with significantly earlier neurologic improvement when compared to the receipt of IV alteplase alone. Patients in the intervention group also achieved greater overall reperfusion after 24 hours, corresponding to improved functional outcomes measured at 90 days. The use of CT perfusion imaging also shortened the time to treatment initiation. The results of this study were echoed in the Endovascular Treatment for Small Core and Anterior Circulation Proximal Occlusion with Emphasis on Minimizing CT to Recanalization Times (ESCAPE) trial published in the same issue of The New England Journal of Medicine (NEJM).

ESCAPE

Like the EXTEND-IA trial, patients in the Endovascular Treatment for Small Core and Anterior Circulation Proximal Occlusion with Emphasis on Minimizing CT to Recanalization Times (ESCAPE) trial were initially evaluated using CT and CTA, and considered eligible if they had a small infarct core, an occluded proximal artery in the anterior circulation, and moderate-to-good collateral circulation. Unlike the ESCAPE trial, however, enrollment up to 12 hours after the onset of stroke symptoms was permitted, and intraarterial therapy was not restricted to the use of retrievable stents. As this study was also terminated early, results reflected that of an interim analysis, where the intervention was significantly favored with respect to improved functional outcomes. The mortality rate among patients that received both intraarterial therapy and IV alteplase was also significantly decreased when compared to patients that received alteplase alone, and rates of symptomatic intracerebral hemorrhage did not significantly differ. The median time from initial imaging to groin puncture and median time to first visualization of reflow in the middle cerebral artery in the intervention group were also considerably reduced compared to previous studies, including the EXTEND-IA trial.

SWIFT-PRIME

Less than six months after the release of the EXTEND-IA and ESCAPE trials, the results of the Solitaire with the Intention for Thrombectomy as Primary Endovascular Treatment (SWIFT PRIME) emerged. Using similar methodology to the EXTEND-IA and ESCAPE studies, namely strict imaging eligibility requirements, Saver and colleagues further confirmed that patients receiving IV t-PA and thrombectomy using a stent retriever had significantly better functional outcomes at 90 days, with the proportion of patients achieving functional independence far exceeding that observed in patients that received t-PA alone. The proportion of patients with successful reperfusion in the intervention group was also twice as high as that seen in the control group, without significantly increasing the risk of serious adverse events or 90-day mortality. This study also noted that patients who received IV t-PA at another hospital before being transferred to a study site for thrombectomy had less favorable outcomes, where levels of functional independence in these patients did not significantly from that observed in patients receiving t-PA alone.

REVASCAT

The Randomized Trial of Revascularization with Solitaire FR Device versus Best Medical Therapy in the Treatment of Acute Stroke Due to Anterior Circulation Large Vessel Occlusion Presenting within Eight Hours of Symptom Onset (REVASCAT) study also reiterated the value of administering combination intraarterial and medical therapy. Like the prior studies, following visualization of an occlusion in the proximal anterior circulation without a large core, patients were randomized to receive thrombectomy using a stent retriever and medical therapy or medical therapy alone. Consistent with the aforementioned studies, patients in the intervention group had significantly improved functional outcomes compared to those that received medical therapy alone. Patients that received intraarterial therapy were also significantly more likely to exhibit dramatic neurologic improvements at 24 hours, without an increase in the risk experiencing serious adverse events or death.

Berkhemer OA, Fransen PSS, Beumer D, van den Berg LA, Lingsma HF, Yoo AJ, et al. A Randomized Trial of Intraarterial Treatment for Acute Ischemic Stroke. The New England Journal of Medicine. 2015 Jan;372(1):11-20.

Campbell BCV, Mitchell PJ, Kleinig TJ, Dewey HM, Churilov L, Yassi N, et al. Endovascular Therapy for Ischemic Stroke with Perfusion-Imaging Selection. The New England Journal of Medicine. 2015 Mar;372(11):1009-18.

Goyal M, Demchuk AM, Menon BK, Eesa M, Rempel JL, Thornton J, et al. Randomized Assessment of Rapid Endovascular Treatment of Ischemic Stroke. The New England Journal of Medicine. 2015 Mar;372(11):1019-30.

Saver JL, Goyal M, Bonafe A, Diener H-C, Levy EI, Pereira VM, et al. Stent-Retriever Thrombectomy after Intravenous t-PA versus t-PA Alone in Stroke. The New England Journal of Medicine. 2015 Jun;372(24):2285-95.

Jovin TG, Chamorro A, Cobo E, de Miquel MA, Molina CA, Rovira A, et al. Thrombectomy within 8 Hours after Symptom Onset in Ischemic Stroke. The New England Journal of Medicine. 2015 Jun;372(24):2296-306.

	Study population	Methodology	Results	Key findings
MR CLEAN (2015)	– Patients ≥18 years of age with proximal arterial occlusion in the anterior circulation established with CTA, magnetic resonance angiography (MRA) or digital-subtraction angiography (DSA) – Patients must have been within 6 hours of symptom onset	– RCT (n=500) – Endovascular therapy (intra-arterial thrombolysis and/or mechanical thrombectomy) and IV t-PA vs. IV t-PA alone – Primary outcome: functional outcome by modified Rankin scale (MRS) at 90 days	– Improved functional outcomes by MRS at 90 days in endovascular group (OR 1.67, 95% CI 1.21-2.30) – 75.4% of intervention group had no intracranial occlusion on follow-up CTA (OR 6.88, 95%CI 4.34-10.94) – No difference in occurrence of serious adverse events ($p = 0.31$) between groups	– Endovascular therapy was associated with improved function outcome compared to IV t-PA alone – No increase in serious adverse events with endovascular therapy
EXTEND-IA (2015)	– Patients with anterior circulation ischemic stroke established with CTA – Patients must have had a dual target of vessel occlusion and evidence of salvageable tissue on perfusion imaging and received IV t-PA within 4.5 hours of symptom onset	– RCT (n=70) – Mechanical thrombectomy and IV t-PA vs. IV t-PA alone – Primary outcome(s): reperfusion (% reduction in perfusion-lesion volume at 24 hours) and early neurologic improvement by NIH stroke scale	– Median % reperfusion at 24 hours in the endovascular group was 100% compared to 37% in IV t-PA only group (OR 4.7, 95% CI 2.5-9.0) – Higher proportion of patients from intervention group achieved early neurologic improvement (OR 6.0, 95% CI 2.0-18.0) – Improved functional outcomes by MRS at 90 days in thrombectomy group (OR 2.0, 95% CI 1.2-3.8)	– Mechanical thrombectomy improved reperfusion, early neurologic recovery and functional outcomes compared to IV t-PA alone – CT perfusion imaging can be used to identify patients with the greatest potential to benefit from endovascular therapy, and shorten time to treatment initiation

ESCAPE (2015)	– Patients ≥18 years of age with a small infarct core, proximal intracranial occlusion in the anterior circulation, and moderate-good collateral circulation by CTA – Patients were enrolled up to 12 hours after symptom onset and must have received IV t-PA within 4.5 hours of symptom onset	– RCT (n=316) – Mechanical thrombectomy and IV t-PA vs. IV t-PA alone – Primary outcome: function outcome by MRS at 90 days	– Improved functional outcomes by MRS at 90 days in thrombectomy group (OR 2.6, 95% CI 1.7-3.8) – Intervention associated with reduced mortality (RR 0.5, 95% CI 0.3-1.0)	– Mechanical thrombectomy was associated with improved functional outcomes and reduced mortality compared to IV t-PA alone
SWIFT PRIME (2015)	– Patients with confirmed occlusions in the proximal anterior intracranial circulation without large ischemic-core lesions detected through imaging – Patients must have been within 6 hours of symptom onset and must have IV t-PA within 4.5 hours of symptom onset	– RCT (n=196) – Mechanical thrombectomy with stent retriever and IV t-PA vs. IV t-PA alone – Primary outcome: functional outcome by MRS at 90 days	– Improved functional outcomes by MRS at 90 days in thrombectomy group ($p<0.001$) – Successful reperfusion (≥90%) at 27 hours was more frequent in the intervention group ($p<0.001$) – No difference in occurrence of serious adverse events ($p = 0.54$)	– Mechanical thrombectomy was associated with improved functional outcomes compared to IV t-PA alone

REVASCAT (2015)	– Patients age 18-85 years with anterior circulation ischemic stroke without evidence of a large ischemic core on imaging – Patients must have been within 8 hours of symptom onset and must have received IV t-PA within 4.5 hours of stroke onset without evidence of revascularization within 30 minutes of t-PA	– RCT (n=206) – Thrombectomy with stent retriever and IV t-PA vs. IV t-PA – Primary outcome: functional outcome by MRS at 90 days	– Improved functional outcomes by MRS at 90 days in thrombectomy group (OR 1.7, 95%CI 1.05-2.8) and dramatic neurologic improvement at 24 hours (OR 5.5, 95% CI 2.9-10.3) – Mortality ($p = 0.60$) and rates of intracranial hemorrhage ($p = 1.00$) did not significantly differ at 90 days	– Mechanical thrombectomy was associated with improved function outcomes, without an increased risk of mortality or intracranial hemorrhage compared to IV t-PA alone

Table I. Key stroke trials.

The DAWN Trial: Thrombectomy between 6 and 24 hours after acute stroke reduces disability

1. Thrombectomy performed between 6 and 24 hours after onset of acute stroke in patients with a mismatch between stroke symptoms and infarct volume results in better disability outcomes compared to standard care alone.

2. Adverse events of intracranial hemorrhage and 90-day mortality do not differ significantly between thrombectomy and standard care-treated patients.

Original Date of Publication: January 2018

Study Rundown: Acute stroke management with thrombectomy aims to increase cerebral perfusion in order to minimize ischemic damage. Prior studies have indicated a clinical advantage to performing thrombectomy within 6 hours of stroke onset, with decreasing clinical benefit as time to thrombectomy increases. After 6 hours from stroke onset relatively fewer studies are available to aid in determining optimal stroke management with thrombectomy. In this study, the DAWN (DWI or CTP Assessment with Clinical Mismatch in the Triage of Wake-Up and Late Presenting Strokes Undergoing Neurointervention with Trevo) trial compares stroke patients with a mismatch between their clinical deficits and infarct volume treated 6 to 24 hours after symptom onset with thrombectomy plus standard care compared to standard care alone. Primary endpoints of disability and functional independence were both improved in the thrombectomy group compared to the standard treatment group at 90 days post treatment. Rates of internal hemorrhage and 90-day mortality did not significantly differ between the two groups.

This study provides significant evidence supporting thrombectomy treatment between 6 and 24 hours after stroke onset. Study strengths include participation of numerous multinational treatment centers and extensive subgroup analysis, and a notable weakness is exclusion of patients with large volume infarcts.

In-Depth [randomized controlled trial]: This prospective, multicenter trial conducted between 2014 and 2017 randomized 206 patients to thrombectomy plus standard care (n = 107) and standard care (n = 99) groups. Eligible patients had occlusion of either the intracranial internal carotid artery, proximal middle cerebral artery, or both with a last known well time between 6 and 24 hours prior to treatment. Included patients also had a mismatch between their clinical symptom severity and infarct volume as defined by the National Institutes of Health Stroke Scale (NIHSS). Concomitant stenting was not performed in the thrombectomy group. The modified Rankin scale was used to assess co-primary endpoints of disability and functional independence.

Patients in the thrombectomy group were less disabled at 90 days post-treatment compared to the standard care group (5.5 vs 3.4 Rankin score, respectively; 95% confidence interval 1.1 to 3.0). Rates of functional independence at 90 days were 49% in the thrombectomy group and 13% in the control group (adjusted difference 33%; 95% credible interval 22 to 40). Subgroup analysis indicated significantly improved disability scores for thrombectomy-treated patients for almost all assessments (except for unwitnessed stroke). Rates of intracerebral hemorrhage (6% vs 3%, p = 0.50) and 90-day mortality (19% vs 18%, p = 1.00) did not differ between the thrombectomy and standard care groups, respectively.

Nogueira RG, Jadhav AP, Haussen DC, Bonafe A, Budzik RF, Bhuva P, et al. Thrombectomy 6 to 24 Hours after Stroke with a Mismatch between Deficit and Infarct. N Engl J Med. 2018 04;378(1):11–21.

The DEFUSE 3 Trial: Thrombectomy improves functional outcomes for imaging screened patients 6 to 16 hours after stroke

1. Patients presenting with ischemic stroke 6 to 16 hours after they were last known to be well had improved functional outcomes at 90 days if treated with thrombectomy and medical therapy compared to medical therapy alone.

2. Mortality at 90 days trended towards a lower rate in the thrombectomy group compared to the medical therapy group.

Original Date of Publication: February 2018

Study Rundown: Patients presenting with ischemic stroke within 6 hours are preferentially treated with endovascular thrombectomy, and recent reports suggest thrombectomy may be beneficial after 6 hours from a patient's last known well time. Additionally, imaging studies can identify patients with ischemic but not infarcted tissue who may benefit from thrombectomy. The DEFUSE 3 (Endovascular Therapy Following Imaging Evaluation for Ischemic Stroke) trial evaluates whether thrombectomy can benefit patients with ischemic stroke from 6 to 16 hours after their last known well time. The trial was stopped early as the primary outcome of a functional disability score at 90 days was significantly better in patients treated with thrombectomy and standard medical care versus medical care alone. The mortality rate trended towards a lower rate in the thrombectomy group, and no differences in intracranial hemorrhage or other adverse events were observed between the two groups.

The study's strengths include participation numerous medical centers and rigorous imaging inclusion criteria, and a limitation is potentially less power for showing a mortality benefit with thrombectomy due to the early study termination.

In-Depth [randomized controlled trial]: This multi-institutional, randomized, controlled trial was conducted between 2016 and 2017. Patients (n = 182) were eligible for inclusion if they were last known well between 6 to 16 hours prior to potential thrombectomy and met multiple imaging criteria such as an ischemic volume of less than 70 mL and had a potentially reversible ischemia volume of 15 mL or more. Imaging was done via CT or MRI utilizing a standard postprocessing software (RAPID). Patients were randomized to receive standard medical care (n = 90) or thrombectomy plus medical care (n = 92), with thrombectomy being performed per the discretion of the operating physician. Follow-up clinical assessment using the modified Rankin scale was performed at 30 and 90 days, with comparison of the groups Rankin score at 90 days being the primary outcome and comparison of functional independence being the secondary outcome.

The trial was halted early, with results indicating better Rankin disability scores in the thrombectomy group compared to the medical therapy group (unadjusted common odds ratio, 2.77; 95% confidence interval [CI], 1.63 to 4.70; $p < 0.001$). Patients were functionally independent at a higher rate in the thrombectomy group compared to the medical therapy group (45% vs 17%, respectively; risk ratio, 2.67; 95% CI, 1.60 to 4.48; $p < 0.001$). Mortality was 14% and 26% in the thrombectomy and medical therapy groups, respectively, at 90 days ($p = 0.05$). Rates of symptomatic intracranial hemorrhage and early neurologic deterioration did not significantly differ between the groups.

Albers GW, Marks MP, Kemp S, Christensen S, Tsai JP, Ortega-Gutierrez S, et al. Thrombectomy for Stroke at 6 to 16 Hours with Selection by Perfusion Imaging. N Engl J *Med. 2018 22;378(8):708–18.*

The EXTEND-IA TNK: Tenecteplase superior to alteplase as neoadjuvant treatment for mechanical thrombectomy

1. When treated with tenecteplase, stroke patients eligible for mechanical thrombectomy had higher rates of reperfusion and superior clinical outcomes at 90 days relative to patients treated with alteplase.

2. There was no evidence that rates of intracerebral hemorrhage were different between the tenecteplase and alteplase groups.

Original Date of Publication: April 2018

Study Rundown: Recombinant tissue plasminogen activator, given as alteplase, has for many years been a cornerstone of acute stroke treatment (See "2015 Intraarterial therapy and t-PA trials: MR-CLEAN, EXTEND-IA, ESCAPE, SWIFT PRIME, REVASCAT"). These patients often receive alteplase, a recombinant tissue plasminogen activator (t-PA), prior to thrombectomy. Tenecteplase is another recombinant t-PA that has greater specificity for fibrin and a longer half-life. It is unclear which recombinant t-PA is superior as bridging therapy prior to mechanical thrombectomy.

This randomized controlled trial enrolled patients with large vessel stroke eligible to undergo thrombectomy and randomized them to pretreatment with tenecteplase or alteplase. The primary outcome was a predetermined degree of reperfusion. A key secondary outcome was clinical outcome assessed by the modified Rankin scale. The investigators found that patients receiving tenecteplase had higher rates of the tissue reperfusion and higher modified Rankin scale scores at 90 days.

Strengths of the study include its randomized, multicenter design. The use of a surrogate outcome as the primary outcome in the study is a weakness, as it may not translate to meaningful clinical outcomes. Furthermore, the trial was powered for noninferiority rather than superiority. Overall, these results support consideration for use of tenecteplase rather than alteplase prior to endovascular thrombectomy.

In-Depth [randomized controlled trial]: This was a phase three, multicenter, blinded randomized controlled trial that enrolled 202 patients (n = 101 in alteplase and tenecteplase groups) between 2015 and 2017 to compare outcomes amongst patients treated with either alteplase or tenecteplase prior to mechanical thrombectomy. Key inclusion criteria included onset of symptoms within 4.5 hours and large-vessel occlusion of either the internal carotid, middle cerebral, or basilar artery. There was no restriction by NIH stroke scale score, but patients with preexisting disability per the modified Rankin scale score were excluded. The primary outcome was reperfusion of greater than 50% of the involved ischemic territory, or absence of thrombus during angiography. Secondary outcomes included score at 90 days on the modified Rankin scale, and early improvement in National Institutes of Health Stroke Scale score (NIHSS) at 24 and 72 hours.

The primary outcome occurred in 22% of tenecteplase and 10% of alteplase patients, respectively. The study arm was noninferior (P = 0.002) and superior (P = 0.02) to the comparator group (adjusted odds ratio [aOR], 2.6; 95% confidence interval [CI], 1.1 to 5.9). The median modified Rankin scale score was was 2 in the tenecteplase group, and 3 in the alteplase group (odds ration [OR], 1.7; 95% CI, 1.0 to 2.8; P = 0.04). Evidence of early neurologic improvement (within 24 or 72 hours) did not meet the threshold or statistical significance (P24 = 0.06, P72 = 0.053). One patient in both the tenecteplase and alteplase group had a symptomatic intracerebral hemorrhage.

Campbell BCV, Mitchell PJ, Churilov L, Yassi N, Kleinig TJ, Dowling RJ, et al. Tenecteplase versus Alteplase before Thrombectomy for Ischemic Stroke. N Engl J Med. 2018 26;378(17):1573–82.

The CARP trial: Preoperative revascularization prior to elective vascular surgery

1. In patients with stable coronary artery disease undergoing elective vascular surgery, preoperative revascularization did not significantly reduce short- or long-term mortality.

2. Patients undergoing revascularization experienced significant time delays prior to surgery.

Original Date of Publication: December 2004

Study Rundown: The Coronary Artery Revascularization Prophylaxis (CARP) trial demonstrated that in patients with stable coronary artery disease undergoing elective vascular surgery, pre-operative coronary revascularization did not provide any benefit in terms of reducing the risk of myocardial infarction or mortality (i.e., short- or long-term). Patients undergoing revascularization, however, waited significantly longer before having surgery compared to individuals who did not undergo revascularization (54 versus 18 days). The findings of this study supported practice guidelines at the time, which recommended that coronary revascularization be reserved for patients with symptomatic coronary artery disease. Given the efficacy of perioperative beta-blockers and statins, medical management may be suitable alternatives to revascularization in patients with asymptomatic coronary artery disease.

In-Depth [randomized controlled trial]: Patients undergoing elective vascular surgery have a high prevalence of coronary artery disease and have high-risk of perioperative cardiac complications. The CARP trial, originally published in 2004 in NEJM, sought to explore the long-term effects of pre-operative coronary revascularization in patients undergoing elective vascular surgery, as retrospective studies until that point had mixed findings. Of the 5859 patients screened, 510 patients were eligible and underwent randomization. Patients were eligible if they were scheduled for elective vascular surgery (i.e., abdominal aortic aneurysm, severe occlusive arterial disease in the legs) and had stenosis of at least 70% in one or more major coronary artery that was suitable for revascularization (i.e., percutaneous intervention - PCI, coronary artery bypass graft - CABG). The primary endpoint was long-term mortality, as determined by follow-up. Of the 258 patients who were randomized to the revascularization group, 59% underwent

PCI, while 41% underwent CABG. The median time from randomization to surgery was 54 days in the revascularization group and 18 days in the non-revascularization group ($p < 0.001$). There were no significant differences between the groups in terms of the incidence of myocardial infarction or death in the 30 days following surgery. There were no significant differences between the two groups in terms of long-term mortality.

McFalls EO, Ward HB, Moritz TE, Goldman S, Krupski WC, Littooy F, et al. Coronary-Artery Revascularization before Elective Major Vascular Surgery. The New England Journal of Medicine. 2004 Dec 30;351(27):2795–804.

The ICTUS trial: Early invasive versus selectively invasive management for acute coronary syndrome

1. There was no significant difference in the composite rate of death, nonfatal myocardial infarction (MI), or rehospitalization for angina in patients with acute coronary syndrome (ACS) treated with early invasive or selectively invasive strategies.

2. Myocardial infarction was significantly more frequent in the early invasive management group but rehospitalization was significantly less frequent in this group.

Original Date of Publication: September 2005

Study Rundown: Guidelines of the American College of Cardiology-American Heart Association and European Society of Cardiology recommend an early invasive strategy for the treatment of ACS without ST-segment elevation. The Invasive versus Conservative Treatment in Unstable Coronary Syndromes (ICTUS) trial suggested that selectively invasive management may be an acceptable alternative approach to treatment. With advances in medical therapy and higher rates of revascularization, patients treated with the selectively invasive strategy showed no difference in the cumulative rate of death, nonfatal MI, or rehospitalization for angina 1 year after randomization. These results suggest that an early invasive strategy may not be superior to a selectively invasive strategy for the treatment of ACS without ST-segment elevation and with elevated cardiac troponin T levels.

In-Depth [randomized controlled trial]: The authors assigned 1200 patients with ACS without ST-segment elevation and with elevated cardiac troponin T levels to management with early invasive strategy or selectively invasive strategies. Both treatment groups received optimized medical therapy. The early invasive strategy involved angiography within 24 to 48 hours of randomization and percutaneous coronary intervention when appropriate. Patients assigned to selectively invasive management were scheduled for angiography and revascularization only if symptoms persisted despite medical therapy or if patients showed hemodynamic or rhythmic instability. A composite of death, recurrent MI or rehospitalization for angina within 1 year was measured as the primary endpoint. There was no significant difference in the cumulative event rate at 1 year between the groups (RR 1.07; 95%CI 0.87-1.33; $p = 0.33$). Mortality 1 year after randomization was 2.5% in both groups. The risk of MI was significantly higher in the early invasive strategy group ($p = 0.005$), while rehospitalization was significantly less frequent in this group ($p = 0.04$).

De Winter RJ, Windhausen F, Cornel JH, Dunselman PHJM, Janus CL, Bendermacher PEF, et al. Early Invasive versus Selectively Invasive Management for Acute Coronary Syndromes. The New England Journal of Medicine. 2005 Sep 15;353(11):1095–104.

The COURAGE trial: Percutaneous coronary intervention does not improve mortality in stable coronary artery disease

1. The addition of percutaneous cutaneous intervention (PCI) to optimal medical therapy for patients with stable coronary artery disease did not improve mortality or cardiovascular outcomes.

Original Date of Publication: April 2007

Study Rundown: The Clinical Outcomes Utilizing Revascularization and Aggressive Drug Evaluation (COURAGE) trial was the first to provide evidence that in patients with stable coronary artery disease, the addition of PCI to optimal medical therapy does not provide any mortality benefit or improve cardiovascular outcomes. A subsequent report from the COURAGE investigators demonstrated that patients who received PCI were free of angina and had improvements in various quality of life parameters at 3 months after the intervention, though this difference was not sustained at 36 months. Optimization of medical therapy alone without PCI is sufficient for initial treatment of patients with stable coronary artery disease. The addition of PCI to optimal medical therapy likely does not improve mortality or cardiovascular outcomes as evidenced by the COURAGE trial.

In-Depth [randomized controlled trial]: A total of 2287 patients with stable coronary artery disease, objective evidence of myocardial ischemia, and significant disease in at least 1 major coronary artery were enrolled in this study. Patients were randomized to 2 groups: 1) optimal medical therapy alone or 2) optimal medical therapy with PCI. All patients were optimized medically on an angiotensin converting enzyme (ACE) inhibitor or angiotensin receptor blocker (ARB), antiplatelet therapy (acetylsalicylic acid or clopidogrel), as well as a combination of beta-blockers, calcium channel blockers and nitrates. All patients also received aggressive lipid optimizing therapy. The primary outcome studied was a composite of death from any cause and non-fatal myocardial infarction. The median follow-up period was 4.6 years. In patients undergoing PCI, 89% achieved clinical success. There was no significant difference in the primary outcome between the groups (HR 1.05; 95%CI 0.87-1.27; $p = 0.62$). Furthermore, rates of hospitalization for acute coronary syndrome were not significantly different between the groups (HR 1.07; 95%CI 0.84-1.37; p =

0.56). The need for subsequent revascularization procedures (PCI or coronary artery bypass graft) was, however, significantly higher in the medical therapy group as compared to the PCI group (32.6% versus 21.1%, $p < 0.001$).

Boden WE, O'Rourke RA, Teo KK, Hartigan PM, Maron DJ, Kostuk WJ, et al. Optimal Medical Therapy with or without PCI for Stable Coronary Disease. The New England Journal of Medicine. 2007 Apr 12;356(15):1503–16.

The SYNTAX trial: Coronary bypass superior to percutaneous coronary intervention for triple-vessel or left main artery disease

1. In severe coronary artery disease, coronary artery bypass graft (CABG) was superior to percutaneous coronary intervention (PCI) in reducing the need for repeat vascularization.

2. This study suggested CABG should remain the standard of care for severe coronary artery disease, despite being associated with a higher risk of stroke.

Original Date of Publication: March 2009

Study Rundown: The Synergy between Percutaneous Coronary Intervention with Taxus and Cardiac Surgery (SYNTAX) trial was the first large, multicenter, randomized controlled trial comparing CABG to PCI in severe coronary artery disease. This non-inferiority trial demonstrated that CABG was superior to PCI in preventing a composite measure of death, and this was driven by a decrease in the need for repeat revascularization. CABG, however, was associated with a significantly higher rate of stroke compared to PCI. Strengths of this study included the fact that it was conducted at 85 centers across North America and Europe and that it assessed all-comers with severe coronary artery disease. Criticisms of the study included the limited follow-up of 12 months and that most study participants were male. Thus, in patients with severe coronary artery disease, the SYNTAX trial suggests that CABG remain the standard of care, given reduced rate of the primary endpoint at the 12-month mark.

In-Depth [randomized controlled trial]: The SYNTAX trial, published in 2009 in NEJM, sought to determine the optimal mode of revascularization, CABG or PCI for patients with severe coronary artery disease; that is, previously untreated triple-vessel or left main artery disease. In this non-inferiority trial, the primary endpoint was a composite of death from any cause, stroke, myocardial infarction, or repeat revascularization in the 12-month period after randomization. A total of 3075 patients were included in the trial. Of these patients, 1800 were randomized to either CABG or PCI. For the other 1275, there was only 1 suitable treatment option, and they were enrolled in registries for either CABG or PCI. The majority of patients studied were male

(78%). There were no significant differences between the groups in terms of preprocedural rates of major adverse cardiac or cerebrovascular events. At 12 months, there was a significantly lower rate of the primary endpoint in the CABG group compared to PCI (12.4% versus 17.8%, $p = 0.002$), which was driven by a significant reduction in the need for repeat revascularization (5.9% versus 13.5%, $p < 0.001$). Notably, when compared to PCI, there was a significantly higher rate of stroke in the CABG group.

Serruys PW, Morice M-C, Kappetein AP, Colombo A, Holmes DR, Mack MJ, et al. Percutaneous Coronary Intervention versus Coronary-Artery Bypass Grafting for Severe Coronary Artery Disease. The New England Journal of Medicine. 2009 Mar 5;360(10):961–72.

The EVAR I trial: Endovascular versus open abdominal aortic aneurysm repair

The Endovascular Aneurysm Repair (EVAR) trials were randomized controlled trials conducted to explore the safety and efficacy of repairing abdominal aortic aneurysms using endovascular methods. Two trials were conducted simultaneously and published in the same issue of The New England Journal of Medicine.

1. The EVAR I trial compared the safety and efficacy of endovascular and open abdominal aortic aneurysm repair.

2. There were no significant differences in all-cause mortality between the 2 groups.

3. The endovascular group experienced significantly higher rates of graft-related complications and reinterventions.

Original Date of Publication: May 2010

Study Rundown: Endovascular aortic aneurysm repair was first introduced in the late 1980s as an alternative for people considered unfit for open surgery. Several randomized controlled trials have demonstrated benefits of endovascular repair with regards to 30-day mortality, and it has become increasingly used to manage patients with abdominal aortic aneurysm. There was, however, a paucity of data with regards to the long-term follow-up of endovascular repairs. The EVAR I trial was a landmark study that compared mortality and graft-related complication/reintervention rates in patients who had undergone endovascular and open aortic aneurysm repairs. There were no significant differences between the 2 groups in terms of all-cause mortality. While early aneurysm-related mortality (i.e., 0-6 months after repair) was significantly lower in the endovascular repair group, this trend reversed in the longer run. More than 4 years after the repair, the endovascular repair group had significantly higher aneurysm-related mortality than the open group. Moreover, there were significantly higher rates of graft-related complications and reinterventions in the endovascular repair group.

In-Depth [randomized controlled trial]: Patients were eligible for the trial if they were at least 60 years of age, had an abdominal aortic aneurysm with a diameter of at least 5.5 cm on computed tomography, and were anatomically and clinically suitable for either endovascular or open repair. Eligible participants were then randomized to receive either endovascular or open aneurysm repair. The primary outcome was all-cause mortality, while other outcomes were aneurysm-related mortality, graft-related complications, and graft-related reinterventions. A total of 1252 patients were recruited for the trial from 37 hospitals across the UK. Approximately 90.7% of the study participants were male. There were no significant differences between the two groups in all-cause mortality at any timepoint. With regards to aneurysm-related mortality, there were significantly fewer deaths in the endovascular repair group until 6 months after the repair (adjusted HR 0.47; 95%CI 0.23-0.93), though this difference was not observed 6 months to 4 years after the repair. More than 4 years after the repair, there were significantly more aneurysm-related deaths in the endovascular groups compared to the open repair group (adjusted HR 4.85; 95%CI 1.04-22.72). There were significantly higher rates of graft-related complications and reinterventions in the endovascular repair group compared to the open group.

The United Kingdom EVAR Trial Investigators. Endovascular versus open repair of abdominal aortic aneurysm. Maedica (Buchar). 2010 Apr;5(2):148.

The EVAR II trial: Endovascular approach when unfit for open aortic aneurysm repair

1. The EVAR II trial compared endovascular abdominal aortic aneurysm repair with no intervention in patients unsuitable for the open procedure.

2. There were significantly fewer aneurysm-related deaths in the endovascular group compared to no intervention.

3. The rates of complication and reintervention were similar to the rates observed in EVAR I.

Original Date of Publication: May 2010

Study Rundown: Endovascular aortic aneurysm repair was first introduced in the late 1980s as an alternative for people considered unfit for open surgery. The purpose of the EVAR II trial was to assess the benefits and risks associated with endovascular aortic aneurysm repair in patients who were unfit for the open procedure. There were no significant differences between the two groups in terms of all-cause mortality, though aneurysm-related mortality was significantly lower in the endovascular repair group. This benefit was largely attributed to the significant reductions observed in the 6-month to 4-year period following the repair procedure. Notably, the graft-related complication and reintervention rates were comparable to those observed in the EVAR I trial.

In-Depth [randomized controlled trial]: The EVAR II trial, originally published in 2010 in NEJM, focused on patients who were physically unsuitable for open abdominal aneurysm repair. The trial was supported by the National Institute for Health Research of the United Kingdom (UK). Patients were eligible for the trial if they were at least 60 years of age and had an abdominal aortic aneurysm with a diameter of at least 5.5 cm on computed tomography. Moreover, eligible patients were unsuitable for open repair, but candidates for endovascular repair. Eligible participants were then randomized to receive either endovascular aneurysm repair or no intervention. Again, the primary outcome was all-cause mortality, while other outcomes were aneurysm-related mortality, graft-related complications, and graft-related reinterventions. A total of 404 patients were recruited from 33 different hospitals across the UK. Approximately 86% of the participants were male. With regards to all-cause mortality, there were no significant differences between the two groups at any timepoint following the repair. Notably, there were significantly fewer aneurysm-related deaths in the endovascular group compared to the no intervention group (adjusted HR 0.53; 95%CI 0.32-0.89). This difference was driven by significant reductions in mortality in the 6-month to 4-year period following repair (adjusted HR 0.34; 95%CI 0.16-0.72). In total, 158 graft-related complications and 66 graft-related interventions were observed during the trial, and these rates were comparable to the rates observed in the EVAR I trial.

United Kingdom EVAR Trial Investigators, Greenhalgh RM, Brown LC, Powell JT, Thompson SG, Epstein D. Endovascular repair of aortic aneurysm in patients physically ineligible for open repair. The New England Journal of Medicine. 2010 May 20;362(20):1872–80.

The RIVAL trial: Radial versus femoral artery access for percutaneous coronary intervention

1. The composite outcome of death, myocardial infarction (MI), stroke, and non-coronary artery bypass graft-related major bleeding did not differ between radial and femoral access for percutaneous coronary intervention (PCI).

2. Radial artery access was associated with a significantly lower rate of vascular complications when compared to femoral access.

Original Date of Publication: April 2011

Study Rundown: For patients with acute coronary syndromes (ACS), vascular access for PCI via the femoral artery is associated with a substantial risk of bleeding, particularly at the access site. Vascular access via the radial artery may reduce bleeding risks since the site is more superficial and compressible. Observational studies suggested that radial access may also be associated with a lower risk of death and MI. The Radial Versus Femoral (RIVAL) trial was the first large, randomized, controlled trial that compared radial access for PCI to femoral access. Results revealed that radial and femoral access did not differ in the rate of the composite primary outcome, which consisted of death, MI, stroke, and non-coronary artery bypass graft (CABG)-related major bleeding. Vascular access site complications, however, were significantly reduced with radial access compared to femoral. In particular, radial access was associated with a decreased risk of developing large hematomas and pseudoaneurysms requiring closure. Finally, there was a significant interaction between the primary outcome and the volume of radial PCIs performed by the medical center. One potential limitation of the study was the overall low rate of major bleeding, which may have prevented the detection of a significant difference in non-CABG-related bleeding due to radial versus femoral access. This may have been due to the study's use of experienced, high-volume interventional cardiologists whose technical skills may be superior to those of other cardiologists. In summary, the RIVAL trial demonstrated that radial and femoral artery access for PCI are equally effective in managing ACS. Radial access, while potentially more difficult to establish, may be preferable due to the significantly lower risk of vascular complications, as compared with femoral access.

In-Depth [randomized controlled trial]: The RIVAL trial was a randomized, parallel group, multicenter trial. A total of 7021 patients were enrolled in the trial and underwent randomization. Patients were eligible if they had a diagnosis of ACS and were planning to undergo PCI. Patients were excluded if they presented in cardiogenic shock, had peripheral vascular disease, or a history of previous CABG surgery. Recruited cardiologists were required to have expertise in both radial and femoral artery access, including at least 50 radial procedures. In the end, 3507 participants were randomized to radial access and 3514 participants were randomized to femoral access. The primary outcome was a composite of death, MI, stroke, and non-CABG-related major bleeding at 30 days. There was no difference in the occurrence of the primary outcome between the radial and femoral groups (HR 0.92; 95%CI 0.72-1.17). There was an observed interaction between the primary outcome and a medical center's volume of radial access (HR 0.49, 95%CI 0.28-0.87). Radial access was associated with significantly fewer vascular complications, including development of large hematoma (HR 0.40; 95%CI 0.28-0.57) and pseudoaneurysm needing closure (HR 0.30; 95%CI 0.13-0.71).

Jolly SS, Yusuf S, Cairns J, Niemelä K, Xavier D, Widimsky P, et al. Radial versus femoral access for coronary angiography and intervention in patients with acute coronary syndromes (RIVAL): a randomised, parallel group, multicentre trial. The Lancet. 2011 Apr 23;377(9775):1409–20.

Endoscopic biliary drainage in acute cholangitis

1. For patients with severe acute cholangitis due to choledocholithiasis, endoscopic biliary drainage reduced hospital mortality compared to surgical decompression.

2. Endoscopic biliary drainage was associated with fewer post-treatment complications, although the decrease was not statistically significant for all types of complications.

Original Date of Publication: June 1992

Study Rundown: At the time of this study, surgical decompression was the conventional treatment for severe acute cholangitis arising from choledocholithiasis. Surgery, however, was associated with significant morbidity and mortality. Several uncontrolled studies had shown that endoscopic biliary drainage was a safe therapeutic alternative for acute cholangitis that reduced the mortality rate. This study was the first randomized, controlled trial that sought to determine the benefits of endoscopic biliary drainage compared to surgical decompression for patients with severe acute cholangitis. Results demonstrated that endoscopic biliary drainage was associated with significantly lowered hospital mortality rates compared to surgical decompression. Endoscopic intervention also significantly reduced the rates of certain complications, including the rates of ventilator support and residual stones after procedure.

A potential study limitation was that patients randomized to receive surgical decompression experienced longer wait times before undergoing treatment compared to patients randomized to receive endoscopic biliary drainage. The treatment delay for the surgery group, on the order of a couple hours, was due in part to the limited number of immediately available operating rooms. This delay could have resulted in worsened cholangitis in the surgery group specifically, and may have potentially biased the study's results in favor of endoscopic biliary drainage. However, these delays reflect the challenges in arranging emergent surgery that occur in practice. In summary, the findings of this study support the use of endoscopic biliary drainage as a safe and effective treatment for severe acute cholangitis due to choledocholithiasis.

In-Depth [randomized controlled trial]: This trial enrolled 82 patients from the Queen Mary Hospital in Hong Kong. Eligible patients included those diagnosed with acute cholangitis due to choledocholithiasis based on the presence of septic shock or progressive biliary sepsis manifesting as mental confusion or antibiotic-refractory fever. All patients underwent emergency diagnostic endoscopic retrograde cholangiopancreatography (ERCP) prior to randomization for endoscopic biliary drainage or surgical decompression. A total of 41 patients were randomized to each treatment group. All patients received definitive therapy following biliary drainage. Mortality was defined as death within 48 hours after biliary drainage, in the absence of other contributory causes. Morbidity included any complications that arose after treatment. Cholangitis was considered to have resolved once body temperature and blood pressure were normalized for at least 8 hours.

The mortality rate was significantly lower for patients undergoing endoscopic biliary drainage compared to patients undergoing surgical decompression (10% versus 32%; $p < 0.03$). The rate of complications was not significantly different between the groups (34% versus 66%; $p > 0.05$). Only the rates of residual calculi and ventilator support were significantly lower for patients receiving endoscopic drainage compared to surgery. The time needed to normalize body temperature and blood pressure was not different between patients receiving endoscopic biliary drainage and surgical decompression.

Lai ECS, Mok FPT, Tan ESY, Lo C, Fan S, You K, et al. Endoscopic Biliary Drainage for Severe Acute Cholangitis. The New England Journal of Medicine. 1992 Jun 11;326(24):1582–6.

Transjugular intrahepatic portosystemic shunt effective in preventing recurrent variceal hemorrhage

1. In patients with recurrent variceal bleeding secondary to portal hypertension, the use of transjugular intrahepatic portosystemic shunt (TIPS) demonstrated high efficacy in preventing variceal re-bleeds.

2. The major complications associated with TIPS are stent occlusion and stenosis as well as an increased incidence of hepatic encephalopathy.

Original Date of Publication: January 1994

Study Rundown: In patients with advanced liver disease and cirrhosis, variceal bleeding resulting from increased portal pressure is a potentially-life threatening complication. Each variceal bleeding episode is associated with a 30% mortality rate and a 70% risk of recurrent bleeding within 1 year. In patients refractory to medical and endoscopic management, surgical portacaval shunts were historically the mainstay of therapy in selected patients. The advent of TIPS, which involves creating a low-resistance channel between the hepatic and portal vein via percutaneous vascular access, provided a less invasive alternative to reducing portal hypertension. The purpose of this landmark prospective trial was to report the safety and efficacy of TIPS in the treatment of recurrent variceal bleeds secondary to liver cirrhosis.

The prospective trial reported the outcomes of 100 patients with cirrhosis and recurrent variceal bleeding. The majority of patients had failed previous endoscopic sclerotherapy. Outcomes of interest included frequency of technical success, evidence of decreased portal pressure via duplex sonography, variceal re-bleeding rates post-procedure, and rates of complication. At the conclusion of the trial, TIPS was successfully performed in nearly all patients in the cohort resulting in a significant reduction of portal venous pressure gradient. Subsequently, over 90% of patients were free of variceal bleeds at 6-month follow-up. The major complications included stent restenosis and occlusion, which occurred in 30% of patients. All patients experiencing complications were successfully managed with re-stent or dilatation. TIPS was associated with an increase in hepatic encephalopathy, although this was comparable to the rates observed in surgical shunts. This trial is limited by the observational nature of the trial and the lack of comparison groups to endoscopic sclerotherapy or surgical shunts. However, this was the first large trial to describe the successful use of TIPS. Future randomized trials have confirmed the conclusions of this trial and have established TIPS as a viable treatment method for patients with recurrent variceal bleeds

In-Depth [prospective cohort]: This was a prospective study of 112 consecutive patients that underwent TIPS for recurrent variceal bleeding secondary to liver cirrhosis. Twelve patients were excluded due to the presence of either portal vein thrombosis, severe hepatic encephalopathy, stenosis of celiac trunk, or another primary liver malignancy. Overall, 90 patients in the cohort had TIPS inserted electively while 10 patients were treated emergently for acute variceal bleeds. The majority (92%) of patients had previous unsuccessful endoscopic sclerotherapy treatment. After insertion of TIPS, patients were followed at 1-month and then at 3-month intervals for sonographic assessment of stent patency and clinical assessment of hepatic encephalopathy. At the conclusion of the trial, TIPS were successfully inserted in 93 of 100 patients in the cohort. The mean duration of each procedure was 1.2 hours (range 30 minutes to 3 hours). There was significant reduction of portal pressure gradient associated with a significant elevation of portal blood flow post-TIPS. Major complications occurred in 15 patients and consisted of intraperitoneal and biliary hemorrhage as well as hematoma of the liver capsule. Two patients had migration of the stent to the pulmonary arteries.

At clinical follow-up, the proportion of patients that remained free of variceal bleeding at 6 months and 1 year post-TIPS was 92% and 85%, respectively. The 1-year survival in this cohort was 85%. The incidence of hepatic encephalopathy increased from 10% to 25% post-treatment. Older patients and larger diameter of shunt used were significantly associated with development of hepatic encephalopathy. Additionally, 31 patients developed stent occlusion or stenosis. Of these, 10 patients developed recurrent variceal bleeding at 1-year follow-up. Smaller stent diameter was a significant risk factor for stent occlusion/stenosis. All patients experiencing stent occlusion/stenosis were successfully treated with re-stent, thrombolysis, or stent dilation.

Rossle M, Haag K, Ochs A, Sellinger M, Noldge G, Perarnau J-M, et al. The Transjugular Intrahepatic Portosystemic Stent-Shunt Procedure for Variceal Bleeding. New England Journal of Medicine. 1994 Jan 20;330(3):165–71.

Uterine artery embolization effective for uterine fibroids

1. Bilateral uterine artery embolization (UAE) was associated with high clinical efficacy in patients with uterine fibroids.

2. Major complications were rare but included endometria ischemia, endometritis, and permanent amenorrhea.

Original Date of Publication: October 1999

Study Rundown: Uterine fibroids are the most common benign pelvic tumor in women, affecting up to 40% of females over the age of 35 in the United States. Historically, definitive management of patients with symptomatic uterine fibroids consisted of surgical intervention with hysterectomy. UAE, which employs an endovascular approach, was developed to provide a uterus-sparing option for patients who either prefer a less invasive approach or are not eligible for surgery. The purpose of this early retrospective study was to evaluate the effectiveness of UAE in the treatment of uterine fibroids.

This retrospective review included 60 consecutive patients that were referred for UAE with polyvinyl alcohol (PVA) particles for treatment of symptomatic fibroids. The primary outcome of interest was clinical and symptomatic improvement post-UAE. Secondary outcomes included post-procedural complications and sonographic evaluation of residual fibroid volume at follow-up. At the conclusion of the trial, 59 of 60 patients underwent successful bilateral UAE. The majority of patients reported either moderate or marked clinical improvement of their previous symptoms by 2 years follow-up. Furthermore, there was an approximately 50% reduction of dominant fibroid volume in this cohort on ultrasound follow-up. There were two cases of treatment failure resulting in hysterectomy. One case demonstrated permanent amenorrhea post UAE. The results of this trial provided evidence for the use of UAE as an effective, minimally invasive treatment modality for symptomatic fibroids. However, the study is limited by a small sample size and lack of a comparison group to myomectomy or hysterectomy. Additional randomized trials have since demonstrated similar efficacy compared to surgical intervention.

In-Depth [retrospective cohort]: This was a retrospective review of 60 consecutive patients (mean age: 43.5; range 27-66) that underwent UAE for symptomatic fibroids at a single institution in the United States. No patients were excluded from the study. With the exception of one patient, all underwent bilateral UAE with permanent PVA. Each patient underwent routine clinical and ultrasound follow-up at regular intervals at 6 weeks, then at 2, 6, 12, 18, and 24 months. The primary outcome of interest was symptomatic improvement as determined by patient-reported abnormal bleeding and pain Likert scale. Secondary outcomes of interest included rates of complications as well as dominant fibroid volume post-procedure. After a mean follow up of 10.2 months, 47 of 54 (87%) patients and 41 of 45 (91%) patients reported either moderate or marked improvement in abnormal bleeding and pain, respectively. Additionally, 92% of patients demonstrated reduction in the dominant fibroid volume with an average volume reduction of 48.8% (range: -522% to 100%). Two patients required an additional embolization procedure due to recanalization; treatment failure occurred in one patient that required hysterectomy. Common post-procedure complications were abdominal pain (100%), fever (34%), and post-embolization syndrome (10%). Significant complications were rare but included moderate groin hematoma (n=1), permanent amenorrhea (n=1), and delayed infection resulting in hysterectomy (n=1). There was no specific report of patient disposition post-procedure, but 22 patients (37%) required same-day hospital admission for pain management. Univariable analysis demonstrated that patients with large fibroid volume reduction on ultrasound ($p < 0.001$) or with a previous history of myomectomy ($p < 0.02$) were less likely to undergo hysterectomy post-UAE. Additionally, younger patients were more likely to experience treatment failure ($p < 0.02$).

Goodwin SC, McLucas B, Lee M, Chen G, Perrella R, Vedantham S, et al. Uterine Artery Embolization for the Treatment of Uterine Leiomyomata Midterm Results. J Vasc Interv Radiol. 1999 Oct;10(9):1159–65.

Arterial chemoembolization improves survival in non-resectable hepatocellular carcinoma

1. In patients with nonresectable hepatocellular carcinoma (HCC), arterial chemoembolization with doxorubicin demonstrated significant survival benefit compared to control group.

2. The randomized controlled trial had strict inclusion criteria and only included patients with Child-Pugh Class A/B and no evidence of end-stage tumoral disease, portal vein obstruction, or encephalopathy.

Original Date of Publication: May 2002

Study Rundown: HCC is the most common primary liver cancer and the second-leading cause of cancer mortality worldwide. While the mainstay of treatment is surgical resection, many patients do not meet the eligibility criteria for curative resection due to large disease burden. Alternative treatment modalities for patients with nonresectable HCC such as arterial chemoembolization of the feeding hepatic artery were developed; however, early trials evaluating the use of arterial chemoembolization demonstrated conflicting evidence on the survival benefit of these procedures.

The purpose of this landmark randomized controlled trial was to determine the effectiveness of arterial chemoembolization in a study population most likely to benefit from this procedure. The trial randomized over 100 patients with non-resectable HCC to chemoembolization with doxorubicin or symptomatic control. The trial excluded all patients with advanced disease (Child-Pugh Class C), extra-hepatic disease, or portal vein thrombosis. The trial was stopped early due to the significant survival benefit observed in the patient group randomized to arterial chemoembolization. Additionally, the use of chemoembolization was associated with a significantly lower rate of tumor invasion of portal vein at two years of follow-up. The results of this trial demonstrated a significant survival benefit of arterial chemoembolization in a stringently selected patient population with non-resectable HCC.

In-Depth [randomized controlled trial]: This was a single-blind, multi-center randomized controlled trial evaluating the survival benefit of arterial chemoembolization in patients with non-resectable HCC. All adult patients (n=903) with a biopsy- or imaging-confirmed diagnosis of HCC were consecutively screened for enrollment over four years across three centers in Barcelona, Spain. The inclusion criteria were patients with HCC that were deemed not suitable for curative treatment. Key exclusion criteria included patients with Child-Pugh Class C disease, evidence of extra-hepatic disease, presence of vascular invasion, renal failure, or end-stage tumoral disease. Overall, 112 patients with nonresectable HCC were recruited and randomized to either chemoembolization with gelatin sponge and doxorubicin, arterial embolization alone, or symptomatic treatment. Arterial embolization with or without doxorubicin was performed at baseline, 2 months, 6 months, and every 6 months thereafter. Treatment was halted if the patient developed any of the exclusion criteria. Treatment response was monitored by contrast-enhanced spiral computed tomography at 6 months post-recruitment. The primary endpoint was overall survival with a secondary endpoint of treatment response.

Overall, 40 patients were randomized to chemoembolization, 37 patients were randomized to arterial embolization only, and 35 patients were randomized to symptomatic treatment. There were no significant differences in the baseline characteristics between each group with the exception of serum bilirubin, which was significant higher in the control group. The trial was stopped early due to significant survival benefit in the chemoembolization group compared to control (HR: 0.47; 95%CI 0.25-0.91; $p = 0.025$). At the conclusion of the trial, the mean survival for the chemoembolization group was significantly longer compared to control group (25.3 months versus 17.9 months; $p < 0.009$). There were no direct survival comparisons between the chemoembolization group and the embolization group; however, only chemoembolization was associated with a decreased risk of portal-vein thrombosis compared to control at two-year follow-up (17% versus 58%; $p = 0.005$). The mean number of chemoembolization treatment sessions was 3.08 (95%CI: 2.4-3.5). Eleven patients had treatment-related complications and there was one treatment-related death. Common complications included cholecystitis, leukopenia, and spontaneous bacterial peritonitis.

Llovet JM, Real MI, Montaña X, Planas R, Coll S, Aponte J, et al. Arterial embolisation or chemoembolisation versus symptomatic treatment in patients with unresectable hepatocellular carcinoma: a randomised controlled trial. The Lancet. 2002 May 18;359(9319):1734–9.

Percutaneous radiofrequency ablation effective in small, exophytic renal cell carcinoma

1. Percutaneous radiofrequency ablation (RFA) demonstrated high efficacy and safety in patients with exophytic renal cell carcinoma (RCC) tumors up to 5 cm.

2. Large RCC tumors with central renal sinus involvement were associated with increased treatment failure.

Original Date of Publication: February 2003

Study Rundown: RCC is the most common primary kidney malignancy and results in approximately 14 000 deaths annually in the United States. Historically, definitive management of RCC consisted of invasive surgery with radical or partial nephrectomy. Non-invasive management options, including RFA, are alternative modalities for treatment of RCC for patients ineligible for surgical intervention or with the need for nephron-sparing therapy. The purpose of this landmark prospective trial was to report the effectiveness of and to delineate the tumor characteristic most amenable to RFA.

This trial reported the results of 34 patients that underwent RFA for treatment of RCC. The primary outcome was evidence of technical success, which was demonstrated by lack of active disease on follow-up imaging. At the conclusion of the study, all exophytic RCC tumors were successfully treated, regardless of size. The majority of tumors that underwent successful treatment required only one RFA session; large tumors (>3 cm) were associated with multiple ablation sessions. Additionally, large tumors that demonstrated involvement of the central renal sinus were associated with an increased incidence of treatment failure. There were no cases of locally recurrent disease or development of metastatic disease in patients with successful RFA treatment. Complications occurred in a small number of patients, with no cases of death or dialysis requirement due to RFA. The trial was limited by a small sample size and did not include any data for small (<3 cm) tumors with renal sinus involvement. However, this prospective trial demonstrated the effectiveness of using RFA in RCC up to 5 cm in size and not involving the renal pelvis.

In-Depth [prospective cohort]: This was a prospective, single center trial analyzed the results of 34 consecutive patients with biopsy-confirmed RCC that underwent RFA in the United States. Inclusion criteria included ineligibility for surgery due to medical comorbidities, life expectancy >1 year, and presence of solitary kidney. Patients were excluded if there was a lack of a safe percutaneous path for tumor access on imaging. The primary outcome was overall treatment success, which was defined as the absence of enhancement in the area of the tumor on 1-month follow-up imaging. Each RCC tumor was characterized with contrast-enhanced CT scan to determine size and location within the kidney. Tumors with extension into the peri-renal fat space with no involvement of the renal sinus were categorized as exophytic. Additionally, tumors greater than 3 cm in cross-sectional diameter were categorized as large. Overall, 42 tumors from 34 patients underwent RFA. All exophytic RCC tumors (n=29) had a technically successful ablation, regardless of size. Successful ablation was achieved for size as large as 5 cm in diameter. The majority of small (89%) and large (70%) exophytic tumors only required a single session ablation therapy. Only 5 out of 12 large RCC tumors with central renal sinus involvement demonstrated successful ablation. There were no small tumors involving the central renal sinus. In univariate analysis, large tumors with involvement of the central renal sinus were a significant negative predictor of treatment success ($p = 0.01$). After a median follow-up of 9.9 months, there was no evidence of imaging recurrence or development of metastatic disease in patients that underwent successful RFA treatment. Four complications occurred in a total of 54 ablation sessions. These included one minor hemorrhage, two major hemorrhages, and one ureteral stricture. No patients required dialysis post-RFA treatment.

Gervais DA, McGovern FJ, Arellano RS, McDougal WS, Mueller PR. Renal Cell Carcinoma: Clinical Experience and Technical Success with Radio-frequency Ablation of 42 Tumors. Radiology. 2003 Feb 1;226(2):417–24.

Radiofrequency thermal ablation superior to percutaneous ethanol injection in hepatocellular carcinoma

1. In patients with hepatocellular carcinoma (HCC) not eligible for surgical resection, the use of radiofrequency thermal ablation (RFA) demonstrated significantly higher local recurrence-free survival compared to percutaneous ethanol injection (PEI).

Original Date of Publication: July 2003

Study Rundown: HCC is the second-leading cause of cancer mortality worldwide and often occurs in the setting of cirrhosis and chronic liver disease. Curative treatment can be obtained with surgical resection or liver transplantation; however, a large proportion of patients are poor candidates for curative treatment due to poor underlying liver function. Both PEI and RFA are alternative modalities that induce local tumor necrosis in patients with HCC with underlying cirrhosis who are not eligible for surgical intervention. The purpose of this randomized controlled trial was to compare the effectiveness of PEI and RFA in patients with HCC.

The trial randomized over 100 patients with HCC ineligible for surgical resection or liver transplantation to either RFA or PEI, both performed with ultrasound guidance. Patients were excluded if they had advanced liver disease (Child Pugh Class C) or evidence of extra-hepatic disease or vascular invasion. At the conclusion of the trial, there was a significantly higher rate of local recurrence-free survival at 1- and 2-years in the RFA group compared to PEI. Additionally, there was a trend towards the RFA group for improved overall survival, which did not reach statistical significance. The mean number of treatment sessions was significantly lower in the RFA group with no significant increase in the complication rate compared to PEI. The results of this study demonstrate a superiority of RFA compared to PEI and support the use of RFA as the optimal alternative modality in HCC patients ineligible for curative surgical intervention. However, this study does not provide data for survival beyond two-year follow-up.

In-Depth [randomized controlled trial]: This was an open-labeled, multi-center randomized controlled trial analyzing the effectiveness of RFA to PEI in patients with HCC not eligible for curative surgical interventions. The inclusion criteria included all adult patients with cirrhosis and a concurrent single HCC <5 cm in diameter or as many as 3 HCCs with a maximum dimension of <3 cm in diameter. Patients must have been ineligible for surgical intervention or liver transplantation. Key exclusion criteria included presence of extrahepatic disease or evidence of tumor vascular invasion. Patients were also excluded if the HCCs were located less than 1 cm away from the hepatic hilum or gallbladder. The primary outcome was overall survival with a secondary endpoint of local recurrence-free survival rate. Each RFA or PEI procedure was standardized and supervised by a trial co-investigator. Follow-up for evaluation of local recurrence was done by serum α_1-fetoprotein and abdominal ultrasound at three-month intervals and dual phase spiral computed tomography at 6-month intervals.

Overall, 50 patients were randomized to the PEI group and 52 patients were randomized to the RFA group. There were no statistically significant differences in baseline characteristics in each treatment group, with the exception of patient age and albumin concentration. Patients were followed up for mean period of 22.9 months and 22.4 months for the RFA and PEI group, respectively. At the conclusion of the trial, the 1- and 2-year local recurrence survival rate was significantly higher in the RFA group compared to the PEI group (RR: 0.17; 95%CI 0.06-0.51; $p = 0.002$). There was a trend towards increased 1- and 2-year overall survival in the RFA group compared to PEI, which did not reach statistical significance (RR: 0.20; 95%CI 0.02-1.69; $p = 0.138$). Patients in the PEI group had an average of 5.4 (+/- 1.6) PEI sessions while the RFA group had an average of 1.1 (+/- 0.5) sessions. There was no significant difference in the frequency of adverse events such as post-procedural pain and fever. There were no procedure-related deaths, hemorrhage, or infection noted in either treatment group.

Lencioni RA, Allgaier H-P, Cioni D, Olschewski M, Deibert P, Crocetti L, et al. Small Hepatocellular Carcinoma in Cirrhosis: Randomized Comparison of Radio-frequency Thermal Ablation versus Percutaneous Ethanol Injection. Radiology. 2003 Jul 1;228(1):235–40.

The PANTER trial: Open necrosectomy versus step-up approach for necrotizing pancreatitis

1. A minimally invasive step-up approach was associated with significantly reduced rates of major complications as compared to open necrosectomy in patients with necrotizing pancreatitis.

Original Date of Publication: April 2010

Study Rundown: Necrotizing pancreatitis with infected necrotic tissue is associated with high rates of both complication and death. Though first-line treatment is open necrosectomy, this study compared this with a minimally invasive step-up approach, consisting of percutaneous drainage, endoscopic drainage, and/or minimally invasive retroperitoneal necrosectomy. The incidence of multiple organ failure was significantly lower in patients who underwent the step-up approach compared with those who had open necrosectomy. Though the rate of death did not differ significantly between the two groups, patients who were assigned to the step-up approach faced significantly lower rates of both incisional hernias and new-onset diabetes. One limitation of the study was that it was not powered to detect significant differences in death between the 2 groups.

In-Depth [randomized controlled trial]: Originally published in NEJM in 2010, this multicenter, randomized, controlled study involved 88 patients with acute pancreatitis and pancreatic necrosis. They were randomized to receive treatment with either open necrosectomy or a step-up approach, which included percutaneous or endoscopic drainage, and minimally invasive retroperitoneal necrosectomy. The primary end point was a composite of complications (i.e., new-onset multiple-organ failure, multiple systemic complications, bleeding, perforation of a visceral organ) and death. Patients managed using the step-up approach experienced a significantly lower rate of the composite primary endpoint compared to those treated with open necrosectomy (RR 0.57; 95%CI 0.38-0.87). This was largely driven by a significant reduction in new-onset organ failure (12% versus 40%, $p = 0.002$), as there was no significant difference between the two groups in mortality. After 6 months of follow-up, patients who underwent open necrosectomy had a higher rate of incisional hernias (RR 0.29; 95%CI 0.09-0.95), new-onset diabetes (RR 0.43; 95%CI 0.20-0.94) and use of pancreatic enzymes (RR 0.21; 95%CI 0.07-0.67) when compared to those treated with the step-up approach. The study suggests that when treating necrotizing pancreatitis patients, a minimally invasive step-up approach reduces the rate of major complications and long-term complications when compared to open necrosectomy.

van Santvoort HC, Besselink MG, Bakker OJ, Hofker HS, Boermeester MA, Dejong CH, et al. A Step-up Approach or Open Necrosectomy for Necrotizing Pancreatitis. The New England Journal of Medicine. 2010 Apr 22;362(16):1491–502.

Early TIPS in cirrhosis and variceal bleeding

1. In patients with severe liver disease and variceal bleeding, early transjugular intrahepatic portosystemic shunt (TIPS) significantly reduced rates of treatment failure, length of hospitalization, and mortality compared to control.

2. There were no significant differences between the two groups in the rates of adverse events.

Original Date of Publication: June 2010

Study Rundown: Variceal bleeding is a major cause of death for patients with liver cirrhosis and portal hypertension. Guidelines at the time of this study recommended treatment consisting of vasoactive drugs (e.g., octreotide), prophylactic antibiotics, and endoscopic techniques such as variceal ligation for dealing with variceal bleeding. When standard treatment failed, TIPS had been shown to be effective, though was associated with substantial mortality due in large part to hepatic encephalopathy. Previous studies suggested that the earlier use of TIPS can decrease mortality for patients with severe liver disease who are at a high risk of treatment failure. This trial was the first to compare the use of early TIPS with the current standard of care for acute variceal bleeding.

Results showed that early use of TIPS was associated with a significant decrease in the rate of rebleeding and failure to control bleeding. Early TIPS also significantly reduced mortality and led to shorter stays in the intensive care unit (ICU). Notably, early TIPS use was not associated with a significantly higher rate of adverse events, such as hepatic encephalopathy. A major limitation of the study was its small size (only 63 patients were randomized), meaning it was insufficiently powered for subgroup analyses. Thus, for example, the study could not determine whether early TIPS had greater benefit for the study's more severe cases of liver disease (those classified as Child-Pugh Class C) in comparison to the study's less severe cases (those classified as Child-Pugh Class B). In summary, results of this study supported the early use of TIPS for the treatment of patients with severe liver disease and variceal bleeding. Importantly, the results suggested that use of early TIPS was not associated with an increased risk of hepatic encephalopathy.

In-Depth [randomized controlled trial]: Sixty-three patients from 9 centers in Europe were enrolled in this trial. Eligible patients had liver disease classified as Child-Pugh Class B (i.e., moderately severe) or Class C (i.e., most severe), had liver cirrhosis with acute bleeding of esophageal varices, and were already receiving treatment in the form of vasoactive drugs (e.g., octreotide), antibiotics, and endoscopic band ligation (EBL). Patients with age > 75 years, pregnancy, hepatocellular carcinoma, previous TIPS, portal-vein thrombosis, or heart failure were excluded. Within 24 hours of admission, 31 patients were randomized to the "early TIPS" group, where they received treatment with a polytetrafluoroethylene-covered stent within 72 hours after randomization. The remaining 32 patients were randomized to the "pharmacotherapy-EBL" group, where they continued to receive vasoactive drug therapy followed treatment with nonspecific beta-blockers (e.g., propranolol and nadolol) and EBL-TIPS was provided as a rescue therapy. The primary endpoint was the composite outcome of failure to control bleeding and the failure to prevent rebleeding in the next year. Secondary endpoints included mortality at 6 weeks and 1 year, the development of sequelae associated with portal hypertension, and the number of days spent in the ICU.

Results demonstrated that 97% of the early-TIPS group avoided occurrence of the primary endpoint, compared to 50% in the pharmacotherapy-EBL group ($p < 0.001$). At 1 year, the survival rate was 86% in the early-TIPS group compared to 61% in the pharmacotherapy-EBL group ($p < 0.001$). Patients in the pharmacotherapy-EBL group spent a higher proportion of their follow-up time in the ICU ($p = 0.01$). There was no difference in the rate of adverse rates for both treatment groups, including for hepatic encephalopathy ($p = 0.13$), and development of ascites ($p = 0.11$).

García-Pagán JC, Caca K, Bureau C, Laleman W, Appenrodt B, Luca A, et al. Early Use of TIPS in Patients with Cirrhosis and Variceal Bleeding. The New England Journal of Medicine. 2010 Jun 24;362(25):2370–9.

IV. Interface Literature

"Science is a field which grows continuously with ever expanding frontiers. Further, it is truly international in scope…Science is a collaborative effort. The combined results of several people working together is often much more effective than could be that of an individual scientist working alone."

- John Bardeen, PhD

The RECIST 1.1 trial: Measuring tumor burden to assess response to therapy

1. Response to tumor therapy can be assessed by defined target lesions from a subset of measurable lesions.

2. Disease can be classified as demonstrating complete response (CR), partial response (PR), progressive disease (PD), or stable disease (SD) based on the radiographic evaluation of target lesions.

Original Date of Publication: January 2009

Study Rundown: The development of anticancer agents has also necessitated adequate methods to measure tumor response to therapy. In 1979, the World Health Organization (WHO) came together and published a set of criteria to standardize the research definitions of tumor response. Subsequently, researchers continued to disagree on certain definitions, including what constituted a measurable lesion, what the minimum size or number of lesions were to be recorded, how to define disease progression, and how to integrate cross-sectional imaging into response evaluation. These limitations led to modifications of the original WHO criteria, but adoption of these modified criteria remained nonuniform amongst researchers. This heterogeneity in the criteria led to development of new guidelines in 2000, described as the Response evaluation criteria in solid tumors (RECIST), which sought to unify and standardize many of the previously addressed limitations, and provide a consistent framework for the further evaluation of anticancer therapies. The original RECIST guidelines established the conditions for a measurable versus non-measurable lesion, the differences between a target and non-target lesion, and the definitions for therapy response, which included CR, PR, SD and PD.

Since the initial RECIST guidelines, subsequent difficulties and challenges were raised with the defined criteria. Specifically, there was disagreement in the maximum number of lesions to assess in order to measure tumor burden response, how to incorporate pathological lymph nodes into the therapy response, the type of confirmation needed for response in different types of trials, defining disease progression and unequivocal progression, and managing the detection of new lesions. These issues led to development of a RECIST working group to update the original guidelines. A combination of researchers, imaging specialist, and statisticians developed a database of prospective data in order to develop revisions of the original guidelines, named RECIST 1.1. These revised guidelines remained tied to the anatomical evaluation of disease rather than newer assessment tools (i.e., functional or hybrid anatomical/functional assessments of disease).

The RECIST 1.1 guidelines incorporated a large prospective dataset from numerous trials and determined that the maximum number of lesions required to assess tumor burden was 5, reduced from a prior maximum of 10, with a maximum of 2 per organ (down from 5 per organ). Additionally, lymph nodes with a short axis of >15 mm were considered pathological and measurable. These could be defined as target lesions and the short axis measurement were included in the sum of lesions in the overall calculation for tumor response. Another revision of the prior guidelines was that randomized studies with a control arm for comparison did not require confirmation of response, as the control arm allowed for a comparative mechanism to measure response to therapy. Conversely, confirmation of progression is required in non-randomized trials in which the objective response rate is the key endpoint. RECIST 1.1 also updated the definition of disease progression. In addition to the original definition of a 20% increase in sum of the target lesions, it now also required a 5 mm absolute increase in the sum of target lesions (to prevent overcalling progression). Unequivocal progression in a patient with non-target and measurable disease was defined as the substantial worsening of non-target disease, despite stable or responsive disease, that would merit discontinuation of therapy. The use of FDG-PET was also addressed, incorporating it in the assessment of disease progression and/or the identification of new disease. Lastly, while CT and MRI could be used for the assessment of disease, ultrasound was excluded for the use of assessing therapy response.

In-Depth [prospective cohort]: This prospective cohort incorporated data from >6500 patients, including simulation studies and literature reviews. This dataset prospectively documented the change in measurements of solid tumors, which included >18 000 target lesions. Using these data, researchers defined a measurable lesion as one that could be accurately measured, and that the measurement taken was the largest dimension in the plane of measurement, with a minimum size of 10 mm by CT scan (obtained by a CT scanner with a slice thickness no greater than 5 mm). Additionally, a 10 mm caliper measurement by clinical exam can be used (when lesions are superficial, such as a skin nodule), or a 20 mm minimum by chest radiograph to measure index lesions. Lymph nodes were defined as pathological when they measured greater than or equal to 15 mm in the short axis (assessed by CT scan with slice thickness no greater than 5 mm). Lesions that did not meet these criteria were deemed non-measurable. Lesions must have measured >20 mm if non-spiral

CT or MRI was used. Lytic bone lesions were confirmed with PET, bone scan, or plain film, but only measured with CT or MRI, and only if they met the prior measurable requirements. Cystic lesions that were thought to represent metastases were measured if they met measurability requirements, but non-cystic lesions were preferred as target lesions. Lesions that have either coalesced into one lesion or broken up into smaller lesions could be measured, but lesions that have broken into smaller ones were treated individually and measured in their respective largest diameters. Lesions that were too small to measure reproducibly but were present on follow up should be assigned a value of 5 mm.

The response to therapy was obtained by assessing the baseline overall tumor burden, and was only be established in patients with at least one measurable lesion. In patients with more than one measurable lesion, a maximum of five measurable target lesions were recorded as representative lesions, with a maximum of two per organ site. RECIST guidelines delineated that these target lesions should be the largest lesions within their respective organs and should have measurements that are reproducible on subsequent measurements. Tumor burden was defined as the sum of the diameters of the target lesions, with the initial measurement taken as the baseline sum diameter. Once target lesions were identified, they should be used in subsequent evaluation studies. All other lesions identified are labeled as non-target lesions.

CR was defined as the disappearance of all target lesions, with the reduction of all pathological lymph nodes to <10 mm. PR was defined as at least a 30% decrease in the sum of the target lesions, in comparison to the baseline sum diameter. PD was defined as a 20% increase in the sum of the diameters in comparison to the smallest sum of diameters with an absolute increase of at least 5 mm. In addition, any new lesion was considered progressive disease. SD was defined as meeting neither the criteria for partial response nor for progressive disease, in comparison to the smallest sum of diameters.

These guidelines allow for the assessment of therapy response in patients undergoing antitumor therapy, but they rely on the assumption that all disease response is manifested as a steady decline in tumor burden. Subsequent research in novel treatment modalities, such as immune therapy, has suggested that positive disease response may not follow a linear decline in tumor burden, but in fact may have a small period of tumor burden increase or even new lesions on a short-term basis. However, with continued therapy, the overall disease burden may improve or continue to be stable over a long period of time, and suggests that the RECIST criteria may not encompass all types of therapy response, in particular with new targeted therapies.

Eisenhauer EA, Therasse P, Bogaerts J, Schwartz LH, Sargent D, Ford R, et al. New response evaluation criteria in solid tumours: Revised RECIST guideline (version 1.1). European Journal of Cancer. 2009 Jan 1;45(2):228–47.

Additional Review:

Therasse P, Arbuck SG, Eisenhauer EA, Wanders J, Kaplan RS, Rubinstein L, et al. New Guidelines to Evaluate the Response to Treatment in Solid Tumors. JNCI J Natl Cancer Inst. 2000 Feb 2;92(3):205–16.

RECIST 1.1	
Response Category	**Definition**
CR	- Resolution of all known disease - Malignant nodes <10 mm
PR	- Measurable target lesions - 30% decrease in the sum of longest diameter - No evidence of progression of other disease
SD	- Nonsufficient shrinkage to qualify of PR OR - Nonsufficient increase to qualify for PD - Reference: smallest sum of diameters
PD	- Measurable target lesions - 20% increase in sum of longest diameter - Minimum absolute increase of 5 mm - Reference: smallest sum in study or appearance of new lesions

Table I. Recist 1.1 criteria. CR = complete response; PR = partial response; SD = stable disease; PD = progressive disease.

- Measurable lesion: longest diameter measurement of tumor lesions ≥10 mm (CT or skin caliper); ≥20 mm if by chest radiograph.
- Measurable node: ≥15 mm in short axis.
- Baseline sum: sum of diameters of target lesions, nodes, and longest diameters of other lesions.
- Disease burden assessed at baseline: measurable target lesions, up to 5 total (2 per organ); other lesions nontarget.

Immune-related response criteria captures tumor response to therapy

1. Immune-related response criteria should be used to capture the effects of immunotherapeutic agents as they more accurately capture the variable antitumor response seen after their use.

2. Ipilimumab monotherapy resulted in distinct response patterns that are not captured by the existing guidelines for tumor response described by Response Evaluation Criteria in Solid Tumors (RECIST) or other similar guidelines.

Original Date of Publication: November 2009

Study Rundown: The development of anticancer therapies spurred the development of novel methods for measuring therapy response. From early World Health Organization (WHO) criteria to more recent RECIST and RECIST 1.1 criteria, the development of a common language for the description of tumor response has been important for clinical and basic research. Importantly, these criteria have also established the guidelines for defining progressive disease (PD). However, the development of immunotherapeutic agents led to the clinical observation that the response criteria delineated by the WHO or RECIST guidelines did not seem to capture the response of these new, targeted therapies. Specifically, the original paradigm defined stable disease (SD) as a subset that had either not reached a definition for partial response (PR) or PD, and importantly, it was not viewed as an endpoint indicative of therapy response. In the immunotherapy trials however, stable disease has been used as a marker for improved clinical outcome. Another key difference observed in immunotherapy was that patients would often experience an increase in tumor burden before seeing an overall complete response, PR, or SD. Under the RECIST guidelines, a substantial increase in tumor burden would have represented PD, and led to the cessation of therapy, preventing researchers from demonstrating long-term therapeutic effects that may have occurred after this short-term increase in tumor burden.

In 2004 and 2005, an expert panel of over 200 oncologists, immunotherapists, and industry experts convened to develop new guidelines that adequately accounted for these observed clinical differences in patients undergoing immunotherapy. This expert panel used the results obtained from a large clinical trial program of patients with advanced melanoma undergoing immunotherapy. They concluded that the appearance of antitumor activity may take longer for immune therapy than for cytotoxic therapy, and that the response to therapy may occur after PD. They also provided a definition for clinically insignificant PD and suggested that SD durability may represent true antitumor activity. Additionally, new criteria were established for the assessment of tumor response, termed the irRC, which allowed for new lesions to be included into tumor burden without necessarily signaling progressive disease.

In-Depth [expert opinion] An expert panel used the clinical observations obtained from the use of ipilimumab (an immunotherapy agent that directs human monoclonal antibodies to block the CTLA-4 receptor) in patients with advanced melanoma. These clinical observations were obtained from phase II clinical trials that included a total of 487 patients from 3 centers and recorded the patterns of clinical response to immunotherapy. Patients were treated with induction therapy followed by maintenance therapy, and an independent committee used the original WHO criteria and irRC to evaluate tumor response. Patients were expected to experience an increase in tumor burden before a response was obtained, and continued immunotherapy if they had not developed clinical deterioration. About 30% of patients who were treated in the phase II trials had CR, PR, or SD at week 12. Patients with SD at week 12 also demonstrated a slow response (PR and CR) after week 12. Additionally, patients who had PD at week 12 also demonstrated a response to therapy or SD after week 12 with the continuation of immunotherapy. Four distinct patterns of tumor response were obtained: response in baseline lesions by week 12 with no new lesions, stable disease, response after an initial increase in total tumor burden, and a reduction of total tumor burden concurrent with the appearance of new lesions after week 12. WHO or RECIST guidelines had previously not described the latter two criteria.

The irRC guidelines define tumor burden as the sum of diameters of index lesions and of new measurable lesions. Index lesions are defined as the two largest perpendicular diameters of all index lesions (with index lesions defined as up to five lesions per organ, 10 visceral lesions, and five cutaneous lesions). New lesions are limited to those that are greater than 5 mm, up to 5 new lesions per organ, 5 per cutaneous lesions, and 10 visceral lesions. For complete response (irCR), disappearance of a lesions must be confirmed by a consecutive evaluation no less than 4 weeks from the date of first documented complete disappearance. For partial response (irPR), a decrease in tumor burden must be greater than or equal to 50% relative to baseline and confirmed at least 4 weeks after documentation. For stable disease (irSD), response does not meet criteria for irCR or irPR, and there must be no evidence of disease progression. For disease progression (irPD), there must be an increase in tumor burden greater than or equal to 25% relative to the minimum recorded burden and must be confirmed by consecutive assessment at least 4 weeks from the date of first documentation. Patients could have irPR or irSD even in the presence of new lesions as long as they met the definitions of irPR or irSD. These new guidelines for measuring the response to immunotherapies allows for the incorporation of clinical criteria and flexible time points that were previously not captured by the guidelines set forth by RECIST 1.1.

Wolchok JD, Hoos A, O'Day S, Weber JS, Hamid O, Lebbé C, et al. Guidelines for the Evaluation of Immune Therapy Activity in Solid Tumors: Immune-Related Response Criteria. Clin Cancer Res. 2009 Dec 1;15(23):7412–20.

The INVEST: Limited added utility of vertebroplasty versus sham surgery

1. Vertebroplasty does not reduce pain or pain-related disability in patients with osteoporotic compression vertebral body fractures when compared to sham surgery after 1 month.

Original Date of Publication: August 2009

Study Rundown: Osteoporotic fractures of vertebral bodies are often associated with pain and have historically been treated medically, including a combination physical therapy and pain management. These fractures are often a source of pain and disability for patients, and those who fail medical management may require hospitalization or extended care. Percutaneous vertebroplasty, which involves injecting medical cement (polymethylmethacrylate, or PMMA) into the fractured vertebral body, has typically been the next line of therapy in patients who have failed medical management. However, the efficacy of vertebroplasty in relieving pain in osteoporotic fractures has been limited to small case series and nonrandomized controlled studies. Prior to 2009, the best evidence of its efficacy was an open randomized trial involving 34 patients. Despite limited evidence, public institutions have recommended reimbursement for these procedures, which has led to increases in vertebroplasty volume.

The Investigational Vertebroplasty Safety and Efficacy Trial (INVEST) compared the efficacy of PMMA in patients with painful osteoporotic fractures against a sham procedure. The results of this trial showed no significant difference between groups in either the modified Roland-Morris Disability Questionnaire (RDQ) or in pain scores, both measured at 24 hours and 1 month after intervention. These results suggest that there is no added beneficial effect in pain reduction or disability in patients undergoing vertebroplasty for osteoporotic compression fractures. A similar randomized controlled study published concurrently also examined vertebroplasty versus sham surgery, and found no beneficial effect of vertebroplasty at 1 week and up to 6 months after intervention. A Cochrane review confirmed these results in 2015, and concluded that that there was not enough evidence to support vertebroplasty for the treatment of osteoporotic vertebral fractures.

In-Depth [randomized controlled trial]: This prospective trial was conducted at 11 centers across the United States, United Kingdom, and Australia. These sites were chosen because they had established vertebroplasty practices, and a total of 1813 patients were screened for enrollment. Inclusion criteria included patients over the age of 50 that had one to three vertebral body compression fractures (between T4-L5 vertebral bodies) less than one year old who had failed medical therapy. Key exclusion criteria included evidence or suspicion of neoplasm in the target vertebral body, substantial retropulsion of bony fragments, concomitant hip fracture, active infection, uncorrectable bleeding diatheses, surgery within the previous 60 days, lack of access to a telephone, inability to communicate in English, and dementia. The main outcome measures were the modified RDQ and patient rating of average back pain intensity during the preceding 24 hours on a 10-point scale. The minimal amount of change to be clinically significant was 30% in both pain intensity and RDQ. Patients were measured at various points up to one year after intervention, including 3, 14, and 90 days. The vertebroplasty interventionalists had performed a mean of 250 procedures (range of 50-800). All patients who were included in the study underwent fluoroscopically guided infiltration of skin and subcutaneous tissue with lidocaine and infiltration of the pedicle periosteum of the target vertebrae with bupivacaine. Patients were then randomized to either full vertebroplasty or the sham intervention (control procedure). Patients undergoing vertebroplasty had PMMA infused until it reached the posterior aspect of the vertebral body or it entered a paravertebral space. Patients were allowed to cross over to the other procedure 1 month or later after the intervention.

A total of 131 patients with similar baseline characteristics were enrolled between June 2004 and August 2008, with 68 patients who underwent vertebroplasty and 63 who underwent the control sham procedure. There was no significant difference between both groups with regards to either of the primary outcomes at one month. The mean RDQ score (± SD) in the vertebroplasty group was 12.0±6.3 versus 13.0±6.4 in the control group (adjusted treatment effect: 0.7; 95%CI -1.3-2.8; P=0.49). The mean pain-intensity rating was 3.9±2.9 in the vertebroplasty group and 4.6±3.0 in the control group (adjusted treatment effect: 3.9±2.9, CI: -0.3-1.7; P=0.19). Both groups had similar improvement in back related disability 3 days after intervention, which was maintained at 1 month. At 3 months, 9 patients in the vertebroplasty group and 32 patients in the control group had crossed over and underwent the alternative procedure ($p < 0.001$).

Kallmes DF, Comstock BA, Heagerty PJ, Turner JA, Wilson DJ, Diamond TH, et al. A Randomized Trial of Vertebroplasty for Osteoporotic Spinal Fractures. New England Journal of Medicine. 2009 Aug 6;361(6):569–79.

Additional Review:

Buchbinder R, Osborne RH, Ebeling PR, Wark JD, Mitchell P, Wriedt C, et al. A Randomized Trial of Vertebroplasty for Painful Osteoporotic Vertebral Fractures. New England Journal of Medicine. 2009 Aug 6;361(6):557–68.

Vena caval filters in pulmonary embolism prophylaxis

1. Permanent vena caval filter placement in addition to anticoagulant therapy reduced the short-term occurrence of pulmonary embolism (PE), but increased the long-term risk of recurrent deep vein thrombosis (DVT).

2. There was no significant difference in efficacy between low molecular-weight heparin (LMWH) and unfractionated heparin (UFH) as early anticoagulant therapy for PE prophylaxis.

Original Date of Publication: February 1998

Study Rundown: In patients who are at high-risk for PE and have a contraindication to anticoagulation, a vena caval filter is a potential option to reduce the risk of PE. This multicenter study in France is the only randomized, controlled trial that evaluated whether filter placement decreases the incidence of PE, as well as DVT both in short-term and long-term follow-up. The study demonstrated that the use of a permanent vena caval filter in addition to heparin therapy reduced the occurrence of a PE in the short-term. The data, however, also showed that in long-term follow-up of 2 years, there was a significant increase in recurrent DVTs in patients who received a filter. This most likely relates to thrombosis at the filter site, but it may counteract the benefits gained earlier with the reduction in PE occurrence. In summary, this study showed that filters lower the risk of PE in the short-term, but later increase the risk of recurrent DVT. It also confirmed the results of previous studies that showed no difference in effectiveness between LMWH and UFH for early anticoagulant therapy. Overall, the evidence in this study does not support the use of inferior vena cava filters in addition to anticoagulant therapy to prevent PE's and recurrent DVT's. Of note, this study excluded patients with DVT who had a contraindication to anticoagulation, which is one of the commonly cited indications for filter placement.

In-Depth [randomized controlled trial]: This study was a multicenter, non-blinded, 2x2, randomized-controlled trial that randomized 400 patients to vena caval filter placement or no placement, and to receive LMWH or UFH as a bridge to warfarin. Patients over 18 years of age with confirmed DVT with or without concomitant symptomatic PE, and whose physicians believed they were at high risk for a PE, were eligible for the study. Patients with history of IVC filter placement, contraindication to anticoagulant therapy, or likelihood of non-compliance were excluded. Two hundred patients were assigned to receive vena caval filters. One hundred ninety-five of the 400 patients were assigned to LMWH while the other 205 were assigned to UFH for the first 8-12 days of anticoagulant therapy. The subjects underwent a baseline V/Q scan and/or pulmonary angiography to evaluate for a PE. All subjects were transitioned to warfarin therapy after 8-12 days for a duration of 3 months or maintained on UFH if oral anticoagulation was not possible. Patients were followed for 2 years. The primary outcome was occurrence of a symptomatic PE within the first 12 days of anticoagulant therapy. The secondary outcome was occurrence of symptomatic PE, DVT, major filter complication, and/or major bleeding during the follow-up period.

Filter versus No Filter

The study demonstrated that there were significantly fewer patients (2 versus 9 patients) in the filter group compared to the non-filter group who had had a PE in the first 12 days of anticoagulation therapy (OR 0.22; 95%CI 0.05-0.90). Results were similar when analysis was adjusted for heparin therapy and presence of PE at enrollment. In the 2-year follow-up, there was a significantly higher number of recurrent DVTs in the filter group compared to the no-filter group (OR 1.87; 95%CI 1.10-3.20). There was no significant difference in PE incidence, mortality, or major bleeding between the groups at the 2-year mark.

LMWH versus UFH

There was no significant difference in incidence of PE or DVT between the anticoagulant groups during the first 12 days as well as at the 2-year mark. There was also no statistical significance in mortality or adverse effects between the groups. There was no evidence of statistically significant interaction between filter and heparin anticoagulant therapy for both primary and secondary outcome events.

Decousus H, Leizorovicz A, Parent F, Page Y, Tardy B, Girard P, et al. A Clinical Trial of Vena Caval Filters in the Prevention of Pulmonary Embolism in Patients with Proximal Deep-Vein Thrombosis. The New England Journal of Medicine. 1998 Feb 12;338(7):409–16.

The ARMA trial: Lower tidal volume ventilation in acute respiratory distress syndrome

1. This trial was terminated early when the data demonstrated that lower tidal volume ventilator settings in acute lung injury (ALI)/acute respiratory distress syndrome (ARDS) patients reduced in-hospital mortality.

2. Low tidal volume ventilation was also associated with an increase in ventilator-free days and a decrease in the number of days with systemic organ failure. There was no significant difference in the incidence of barotrauma between the low and high tidal volume groups.

3. Patients assigned to lower tidal volume ventilator settings initially required a higher positive end-expiratory pressure (PEEP) to maintain arterial oxygenation and were more likely to develop respiratory acidosis, although the difference disappeared by day 7.

Original Date of Publication: May 2000

Study Rundown: In an effort to maintain normal partial pressure of carbon dioxide and arterial pH, patients with ALI or ARDS requiring mechanical ventilation traditionally received higher tidal volumes (10-15 mL/kg) compared to healthy individuals. However, studies in animals showed that higher tidal volumes were associated with increased lung inflammation and injury. This multi-center, randomized, controlled trial compared traditional tidal volume therapy (12 mL/kg) to low tidal volume therapy (6 mL/kg) in mechanically ventilated patients with ALI/ARDS for 28 days. Results revealed that the traditional tidal volume group had significantly increased in-hospital mortality compared to the low tidal volume group. There was no difference in barotrauma between the groups. In summary, this study demonstrated that lower tidal volumes in ALI/ARDS patients reduced in-hospital mortality and the number of days that patients required mechanical ventilation. Of note, patients in the lower tidal volume group required higher PEEP and had a slight, but significant, respiratory acidosis, both of which resolved after 7 days. This suggested that although lower tidal volumes required a higher respiratory rate to maintain adequate ventilation, its benefits on mortality outweighed the transient acid/base and oxygenation imbalances that were effectively managed with higher PEEP and sodium bicarbonate infusion, respectively.

In-Depth [randomized controlled trial]: This trial was conducted at 10 university centers across the United States from 1996-1999. Eligible patients were above the age of 18, intubated, mechanically ventilated, and had an acute decrease to a P/F ratio (i.e., partial pressure of arterial oxygen to fraction of inspired oxygen) of 300 or less with evidence of bilateral lung edema on recent chest radiograph. Patients with chronic lung disease, high pulmonary capillary wedge pressure or evidence of left atrial hypertension, less than 6 months of estimated survival, and other medical problems that would cause poor respiration or oxygenation were excluded. The authors randomized patients to traditional tidal volume therapy of 12 mL/kg or low tidal volume therapy of 6 mL/kg for 28 days. The investigators tracked patients weekly for a total of 180 days. The primary endpoint was in-hospital mortality, with a significant reduction from 39.8% in the traditional group to 31.0% in the low tidal volume group ($p = 0.007$, 95%CI 2.4-15.3%). There was also a significant decrease in the number of ventilator-free days in the low tidal volume group ($p = 0.007$) and in the number of days free from organ failure ($p = 0.006$).

The Acute Respiratory Distress Syndrome Network. Ventilation with Lower Tidal Volumes as Compared with Traditional Tidal Volumes for Acute Lung Injury and the Acute Respiratory Distress Syndrome. The New England Journal of Medicine. 2000 May 4;342(18):1301–8.

The NETT: Lung-volume-reduction surgery in emphysema

1. Lung-volume-reduction surgery significantly improved exercise capacity, but not overall survival, in patients with emphysema when compared with medical therapy.

2. Post hoc subgroup analyses showed that in patients with upper lobe emphysema and low baseline exercise capacity, lung-volume-reduction surgery significantly decreased mortality compared to medical therapy.

Original Date of Publication: May 2003

Study Rundown: While lung-volume-reduction surgery had been proposed as a treatment option for patients with severe emphysema, there was little evidence examining its effects. The National Emphysema Treatment Trial (NETT) was the first study to assess the morbidity, mortality, and therapeutic benefits of lung-volume-reduction surgery for emphysema patients. The findings of the trial showed that lung reduction significantly improved patients' exercise capacity compared to medical therapy, but did not significantly change overall survival. Post hoc subgroup analyses demonstrated that surgery significantly reduced mortality in patients with upper lobe emphysema and low exercise capacity and significantly increased mortality in patients with non-upper lobe emphysema and high exercise capacity when compared with medical treatment. A major criticism of this trial centers on the survival differences demonstrated in specific subgroups based on post hoc analyses, as opposed to predefined analyses. In summary, results of this study suggest that lung-volume-reduction surgery can significantly improve exercise capacity in patients with emphysema. While subgroup analyses did demonstrate survival benefits in patients with upper-lobe emphysema and low exercise capacity at baseline, these findings should be interpreted with caution given that they were performed post hoc.

In-Depth [randomized controlled trial]: This was a randomized, controlled trial that involved enrollment of 1218 patients from 17 clinics from across the United States. The list of inclusion and exclusion criteria is lengthy - generally, patients were eligible if they had clinical and radiological evidence of emphysema, were non-smokers for at least 4 months, completed all pre-rehabilitation assessments, and were considered fit for surgery. Each patient's distribution of emphysema (i.e., predominantly upper-lobe versus predominantly non-upper-lobe) was determined by high-resolution CT. The primary outcome measures were overall mortality and maximal exercise capacity as measured by cycle ergometry. The secondary outcome measures included pulmonary function, distance walked within 6 minutes, and quality of life, as determined by self-administered questionnaires. Prior to randomization, patients underwent 6-10 weeks of supervised pulmonary rehabilitation. Patients were then randomly assigned to receive lung-volume-reduction surgery (i.e., bilateral stapled wedge resection via median sternotomy or video-assisted thoracic surgery) or medical therapy, and then re-evaluated after 6, 12, and 24 months of follow-up. Improved exercise capacity was defined as a 10 W increase in workload during cycle ergometry.

At 90 days, the mortality rate in the surgery group was significantly higher than the medical therapy group (7.9% versus 1.3%, $p < 0.001$). There was no significant difference in mortality rates when comparing patients who underwent median sternotomy and video-assisted thoracic surgery (8.6% versus 6.1%, respectively, $p = 0.33$). Total mortality rates were not significantly different between the two groups at a mean follow-up of 29.2 months (RR 1.01, $p = 0.90$). Patients receiving surgery had significantly improved exercise capacity as measured by cycle ergometry at 6 (28% versus 4%, $p < 0.001$), 12 (22% versus 5%, $p < 0.001$), and 24 months (15% versus 3%, $p < 0.001$) than the medical-therapy group. Post hoc subgroup analyses revealed that surgery patients with upper-lobe disease and low-exercise capacity had a lower mortality rate (RR 0.47, $p = 0.005$) and experienced significantly improved exercise capacity (30% versus 0%, $p = 0.005$) when compared with similar patients receiving medical therapy only. In patients with non-upper-lobe disease and high baseline exercise capacity, mortality was significantly higher in the surgical group (RR 2.06, $p = 0.02$).

Fishman A, Martinez F, Naunheim K, Piantadosi S, Wise R, Ries A, et al. A randomized trial comparing lung-volume-reduction surgery with medical therapy for severe emphysema. The New England Journal of Medicine. 2003 May 22;348(21):2059–73.

The Wells DVT criteria: A clinical prediction model for deep vein thrombosis

1. The Wells DVT criteria estimated the pre-test probability of deep vein thrombosis (DVT).

2. D-dimer testing in outpatients informed the need for venous ultrasonography in the diagnosis of DVT.

Original Date of Publication: September 2003

Study Rundown: While DVTs most frequently occur in the lower extremities, they may also develop in the upper extremities and other deep veins, such as the portal vein. Patients with DVT often present with pain, swelling, and erythema in the affected extremity. Pulmonary embolism is a concerning and potentially life-threatening complication of DVT, as pieces of thrombus may embolize to the lungs. As a result, patients with DVT are often treated with anticoagulants or, in certain circumstances, mechanical vena caval filters. Originally developed in 1995, the Wells DVT criteria help determine a patient's pre-test probability of having a DVT. These criteria have been subsequently refined and included in an algorithm to guide diagnostic evaluation for DVT using D-dimer testing and venous ultrasonography. This study was published in 2003 and helped elucidate the role of D-dimer in evaluating patients with suspected DVT. The trial found that the D-dimer test had a negative predictive value of 99.1% (95%CI 96.7-99.9) in patients with low pre-test probability of DVT. In patients likely to have a DVT, its negative predictive value was 89.0% (95%CI 80.7-94.6). Thus, D-dimer testing was deemed useful to rule out DVT in patients with low likelihood of thrombus based on clinical assessment.

In-Depth [randomized controlled trial]: In this study, 1096 outpatients who presented with a suspected DVT were first assessed using the clinical model to determine their pre-test probability of DVT (i.e., likely or unlikely). Investigators then randomized patients to the control group (i.e., ultrasonography) or to the intervention group (i.e., D-dimer and ultrasonography). There were no significant differences between the groups in terms of thromboembolic events encountered in follow-up at 3 months. The D-dimer group was associated with significantly lower use of venous ultrasonography, compared to the control group. In patients unlikely to have DVT, the D-dimer test had a negative predictive value of 99.1% (95%CI 96.7-

99.9). In patients likely to have DVT, the D-dimer test had a negative predictive value of 89.0% (95%CI 80.7-94.6).

Wells PS, Anderson DR, Rodger M, Forgie M, Kearon C, Dreyer J, et al. Evaluation of D-Dimer in the Diagnosis of Suspected Deep-Vein Thrombosis. New England Journal of Medicine. 2003 Sep 25;349(13):1227–35.

Criteria	Points
Active cancer	1
Bedridden recently >3 days or major surgery within 4 weeks	1
Calf swelling >3 cm compared to the other leg (measured 10 cm below tibial tuberosity)	1
Collateral (nonvaricose) superficial veins present	1
Entire leg swollen	1
Localized tenderness along deep venous system	1
Pitting edema, greater in symptomatic leg	1
Paralysis, paresis, or recent plaster immobilization of the lower extremity	1
Previously documented DVT	1

Table I. The Wells DVT Criteria. ≥2 indicates that the probability of DVT is likely; <2 indicates that the probability of DVT is unlikely.

Stereotactic body radiotherapy as a state of the art treatment option in inoperable non-small cell lung cancer

1. Stereotactic body radiotherapy (SBRT) achieved a 3-year local tumor control rate of 92% with limited toxicity, making SBRT a valuable treatment option in inoperable (and potentially even operable) patients

Original Date of Publication: July 2009

Study Rundown: Lung cancer is the most common cancer worldwide, and non-small cell lung cancer (NSCLC) accounts for the majority of cases. Surgical resection remains the mainstay of treatment for patients with stage I NSCLC approved for surgery. Historically, medically inoperable patients with NSCLC were managed with radiation therapy (RT) and showed poor five-year survival rates, presumably from insufficient doses. Phase II trials, however, have shown that SBRT – a method using precise targeted radiation to minimize radiation to adjacent tissue – produces tumor control rates even higher than surgical intervention. SBRT can thus administer biologic doses up to twice as high as RT without harmful affects to normal tissue.

Though studies have shown good rates of local tumor control and toxicity for SBRT, the vast majority have been retrospective. Given the paucity of prospective trials and the lack of long-term follow-up data, application of SBRT remains limited. This multicenter prospective phase II study assessed the 36-month survival of NSCLC and evaluated tumor control, survival, and toxicity based on SBRT. The results indicate a tumor control rate similar to surgery in operative cases, a favorable 3-year cancer specific-survival rate, and minimal toxicity. The later Radiation Therapy Oncology Group (RTOG) 0236 trial from Timmerman et al. reported an even high rate of primary tumor control with minimal toxicity. It is noted that the optimal dose and schedule for SBRT is still undefined for treating NSCLC.

In-Depth [prospective cohort]: This prospective phase II study recruited 60 patients with medically inoperable stage I NSCLC, mainly due to COPD (60%) or cardiovascular disease (25%) across 7 centers in Nordic countries. Patients with prior malignancy or a primary tumor next to the trachea, main bronchus, or esophagus were excluded to ensure safety. After patients were referred to RT units, two were excluded based on insufficient radiation dose and one was lost to follow-up. The remaining 57 patients with NSCLC (70% T1N0M0 and 30% T2N0M0) were treated with SBRT using 6 MV from a linear accelerator, after defining the gross tumor volume (GTV, the size of the macroscopic tumor), clinical target volume (CTV, the volume of microscopic and gross malignant tissue), and planning target volume (PTV, the CTV plus a margin of safety around the tumor). CT was performed before each treatment to verify target reproducibility. Patients were then assessed with toxicity grading and chest CT or x-ray at 6 weeks, every 3 months for the first 18 months, and at 24 and 36 months following treatment. Lung function was measured at 3, 9, and 18 months using the Karnofsky performance score.

After the study's conclusion at 36 months, the Kaplan-Meier estimated progression-free survival rate was 52%. The lung cancer-specific survival rates at 1, 2, and 3 years were 93%, 88%, and 88%, respectively. The Kaplan-Meier estimated local tumor control at 3 years was 92%. Four patients (7%), all with T2N0M0 tumors, showed local tumor progression. No patient was lethally affected by SBRT and 14 patients (25%) had no pulmonary adverse effects.

Baumann P, Nyman J, Hoyer M, Wennberg B, Gagliardi G, Lax I, et al. Outcome in a Prospective Phase II Trial of Medically Inoperable Stage I Non–Small-Cell Lung Cancer Patients Treated With Stereotactic Body Radiotherapy. JCO. 2009 Jul 10;27(20):3290–6.

Additional Review:

Timmerman R, Paulus R, Galvin J, Michalski J, Straube W, Bradley J, et al. Stereotactic Body Radiation Therapy for Inoperable Early Stage Lung Cancer. JAMA. 2010 Mar 17;303(11):1070–6.

The PROSEVA trial: Proning in severe ARDS

1. In patients with severe acute respiratory distress syndrome (ARDS), prone-positioning significantly reduced 28- and 90-day mortality when compared to patients who remained in supine position only.

2. **Proned patients were also successfully extubated at higher rates and required fewer days of ventilation when compared to supine patients.**

Original Date of Publication: June 2013

Study Rundown: ARDS is characterized by the 4 following criteria: 1) lung injury of acute onset (i.e., within 1 week of a clinical insult), 2) bilateral opacities on chest imaging, 3) lung infiltrates not cardiogenic in nature, and 4) $PaO_2:FiO_2$ ratio <300. ARDS can be caused by pneumonia, sepsis, blood transfusions, trauma, aspiration, pancreatitis, medications, and chemical inhalation. Previously, the ARMA trial demonstrated that lower tidal volume ventilation significantly reduced in-hospital mortality, while the ACURASYS trial revealed that neuromuscular blockade early in severe ARDS also led to reduced mortality. In the Proning Severe ARDS Patients (PROSEVA) trial, patients with severe ARDS were randomized to either prone-positioning for 16 hours or left in supine position. In summary, proning significantly reduced 28- and 90-day mortality compared to leaving patients in the supine position. Proned patients also experienced significantly higher rates of successful extubation and fewer days requiring ventilation compared to those in the supine group. Notably, all of the centers involved in this study had considerable experience with proning patients.

In-Depth [randomized controlled trial]: This trial was conducted at 27 intensive care units (ICUs) across France and Spain, all of which had at least 5 years of experience with prone positioning. Of the 3449 patients admitted with ARDS, 474 patients were randomized as part of this trial to either sessions consisting of 16 consecutive hours of prone positioning or remaining in the supine position. The inclusion criteria were ARDS (i.e., as defined using the American-European Consensus Conference criteria), endotracheal intubation and mechanical ventilation for ARDS <36 hours, and severe ARDS (i.e., PF ratio <150 mmHg, FiO2 >0.60, PEEP >5 cm H2O, tidal volume 6 mL/kg). The primary endpoint was 28-day mortality, while the secondary endpoints included 90-day mortality, rate of successful extubation, and the number of ventilator-free days.

In the majority of patients, the cause of ARDS was pneumonia. The average number of proning sessions per patient was 4±4, while the mean duration per session was 17±3 hours. All patients in the prone positioning group underwent at least 1 session. The risk of 28-day mortality was significantly lower in patients who underwent proning compared to those who remained in the supine position (aHR 0.42; 95%CI 0.26-0.66). This difference remained significant at 90 days (aHR 0.48; 95%CI 0.32-0.72). Moreover, patients in the prone group experienced significantly higher rates of successful extubation at day 90 (HR 0.45; 95%CI 0.29-0.70) and significantly higher numbers of ventilation-free days at day 28 and 90 ($p < 0.001$ at both time points). With regards to complications, patients in the supine group experienced significantly more cardiac arrests compared to the prone group ($p = 0.02$).

Guérin C, Reignier J, Richard J-C, Beuret P, Gacouin A, Boulain T, et al. Prone Positioning in Severe Acute Respiratory Distress Syndrome. The New England Journal of Medicine. 2013 Jun 6;368(23):2159–68.

Artificial surfactant improves respiratory distress syndrome in infants

1. In 10 infants treated for respiratory distress syndrome (RDS) with artificial surfactant, significant improvements in blood pressure, acid-base status, arterial oxygenation, and radiologic findings were observed.

2. Infants also required significantly less oxygen therapy and ventilator pressure following surfactant administration.

Original Date of Publication: January 1980

Study Rundown: Hyaline membrane disease (HMD), now known as infant RDS, is a pulmonary disease of young infants most often linked to fetal immaturity. After the landmark 1959 discovery by Avery et al. connecting insufficient surfactant with RDS, methods of treating the disease were investigated. As surfactant was known to reduce lung surface tension, making it easier to maintain patent alveoli, this study built upon work in animals as the first trial of artificial surfactant treatment for RDS in human infants.

Using a mixture of natural and synthetic lipids including dipalmitoyl lecithin (the primary component of surfactant) and phosphatidyl glycerol, researchers administered artificial surfactant to 10 infants diagnosed with RDS and examined their laboratory, clinical examination, and radiologic changes. Significant reductions in systolic blood pressure (SBP), along with improvements in arterial oxygenation, arterial-alveolar oxygen concentration differences, acid-base balance, and radiologic findings were observed. Infants also required significantly less inspired oxygen and ventilator pressure after surfactant administration. This study was limited by a lack of randomization, comparison to control infants, and its small sample size. Despite these factors, this study led to future, large, randomized, clinical trials that further solidified the benefits of artificial surfactant use among infants with RDS. Antenatal corticosteroids coupled with post-delivery surfactant and ventilation are now commonplace treatments for infants in neonatal intensive care as they significantly improve clinical outcomes among infants suffering from poor lung development.

In-Depth [prospective cohort]: Ten infants with diagnosed RDS (mean gestational age = 30.2 weeks, mean birthweight = 1552 g) were included in the study. Prior to surfactant administration, ventilator settings were noted and not changed. Arterial oxygen tension (P_aO_2), carbon dioxide tension (P_aCO_2), and pH were recorded 30-90 minutes before and again 10-20 minutes before surfactant administration to provide a snapshot of each infant's physiologic state. No significant differences were noted between these 2 time periods. About 10 mL of artificial surfactant (150 μmol lipid phosphorus/kg) was suspended in normal saline and put into the infants' endotracheal tubes. Infants were then moved into different positions to ensure the solution was distributed to each lung segment and the infant was ventilated with a respirator. Up to 3 hours post-administration P_aO_2, $PaCO_2$, acid-base balance, and radiographic findings were assessed without alteration in ventilator settings. Following this assessment, ability to reduce inspired oxygen concentration (F_iO_2) and respiratory pressure were noted.

On clinical examination, significant increases in SBP post-administration was observed in the 6 infants who had continuous blood pressure monitoring (37 ± 5 mmHg pre versus 59 ± 4 mmHg post, $p < 0.02$). PO_2 increased significantly (45 ± 7 mmHg pre versus 212 ± 46 mmHg post, $p < 0.005$), PCO_2 decreased significantly (50 ± 4 mmHg pre versus 33 ± 2 mm Hg post, $p < 0.005$), and pH increased significantly (7.13 ± 0.05 pre versus 7.31 ± 0.04, $p < 0.05$). Three hours post-administration, F_iO_2 were able to decrease significantly from $81 \pm 7\%$ to $38 \pm 5\%$ ($p < 0.01$) and, within 6 hours of administration, inspiratory pressure could be reduced from 30 ± 2 cm H_2O to 22 ± 2 cm H_2O ($p < 0.02$). The difference in alveolar and arterial O_2 concentration decreased significantly as well 474 ± 49 mmHg to 189 ± 29 ($p < 0.005$) 3 hours post-administration and to 120 ± 18 mmHg ($p < 0.001$) 30 hours post-administration. At an average of 6 hours post-administration complete radiologic resolution of RDS was observed. Two of the 10 infants studied died due to causes unrelated to RDS or surfactant administration. No serious adverse events were linked to surfactant use.

Fujiwara T, Maeta H, Chida S, Morita T, Watabe Y, Abe T. Artificial surfactant therapy in hyaline-membrane disease. The Lancet. 1980 Jan 12;1(8159):55–9.

Additional Review:

Avery M, Mead J. Surface properties in relation to atelectasis and hyaline membrane disease. AMA Am J Dis Child. 1959 May 1;97(51):517–23.

The Lee index: Risk of perioperative cardiac events

1. The Lee index is a prospectively validated model that predicts the risk of a cardiac event in patients undergoing noncardiac surgery.

2. The 6 independent predictors are as follows: 1) high-risk surgery, 2) history of ischemic heart disease, 3) history of congestive heart failure, 4) history of cerebrovascular disease, 5) preoperative treatment with insulin, 6) preoperative serum creatinine >2.0 mg/dL (>177 μmol/L).

Original Date of Publication: September 1999

Study Rundown: Patients undergoing noncardiac surgery are at risk of major cardiovascular complications. With the number of patients undergoing major noncardiac surgery consistently increasing, the incidence of surgery-associated cardiovascular complications has steadily risen. Numerous efforts have been made to identify potential interventions to reduce the likelihood of these complications, with several studies exploring the potential perioperative use of beta-blockers, calcium channel blockers, statins, aspirin, and cardiac revascularization. Several different groups have also attempted to develop tools to stratify patients with regards to their risk of perioperative cardiovascular complications. These include the Kumar, Detsky, and Goldman indices, as well as the American College of Cardiology/American Heart Association algorithm. The Revised Cardiac Risk Index, commonly referred to as the Lee index, was developed by modifying and simplifying the Goldman index. Initially published in 1999, the Lee index is considered the best validated tool for estimating perioperative cardiovascular risk. It uses six equally-weighted criteria to predict the likelihood of a cardiovascular event, and is widely used because of its simplicity.

In-Depth [prospective cohort]: Of the 4315 patients that took part in the study, 2893 were used in the development of the Lee index. The other 1422 patients took part in the prospective validation cohort. The major cardiovascular complications assessed were myocardial infarction, pulmonary edema, ventricular fibrillation/primary cardiac arrest, or complete heart block. Through logistic regression analyses, six predictors of perioperative major cardiovascular complications were identified: 1) high-risk surgery, 2) ischemic heart disease, 3) history of congestive heart failure, 4) history of cerebrovascular disease, 5) insulin therapy for diabetes, and 6) perioperative serum creatinine >2.0 mg/dL (>177 μmol/L). The presence of any of these predictors contributes 1 point to the Lee index score. Higher Lee index scores were associated with higher rates of perioperative cardiac events.

Criteria	Points
High-risk surgery (e.g., emergency surgery, major thoracic procedures, cardiac procedures, aortic/major vascular procedures, procedures >4 hours)	1
Ischemic heart disease	1
History of congestive heart failure	1
History of cerebrovascular disease	1
Insulin therapy for diabetes	1
Perioperative serum creatinine >2.0 mg/dL (>177 µmol/L)	1

Table I. The Lee index.

Lee index score	Derivation cohort	Validation cohort
0	5/1071 (0.5%)	2/488 (0.4%)
1	14/1106 (1.3%)	5/567 (0.9%)
2	18/506 (3.6%)	17/258 (6.6%)
≥3	19/210 (9.1%)	12/109 (11.0%)

Table II. Cardiac event rates based on the Lee index score.

Lee TH, Marcantonio ER, Mangione CM, Thomas EJ, Polanczyk CA, Cook EF, et al. Derivation and Prospective Validation of a Simple Index for Prediction of Cardiac Risk of Major Noncardiac Surgery. Circulation. 1999 Sep 7;100(10):1043–9.

No survival difference in lumpectomy and mastectomy for breast cancer

1. In women with stage I or II breast cancer, there was no significant difference in overall survival in women treated with total mastectomy compared to breast-conserving surgery.

2. Adjuvant radiation therapy was associated with reduced ipsilateral recurrence in lumpectomy-treated women.

Original Date of Publication: October 2002

Study Rundown: Breast cancer is the most common type of cancer affecting women. These cancers arise from tissues in the breast, with the 2 most common types being ductal and lobular carcinomas. Risk factors for developing breast cancer include increasing age, being female, having a family history of breast cancer, certain genetic defects (i.e., BRCA1 and BRCA2), and early menarche/late menopause. While the incidence of breast cancer has increased steadily over the past decades, mortality rates have declined significantly since the 1980s. This may be attributed to increased screening, more effective screening programs, and better treatment amongst numerous other factors. Breast cancer treatment consists of a combination of local and systemic therapy, depending on the cancer characteristics and staging. In the 1970s, several studies were conducted to address lingering questions regarding the surgical management of breast cancer. Several randomized controlled trials were conducted to assess the efficacy of breast-conserving therapy.

This study explored whether lumpectomy, a procedure where the tumor was resected with clean margins, with or without radiation therapy was comparable to radical mastectomy. Previous analyses suggested that there were no significant differences in survival between the study groups. This study reported the 20-year findings of this randomized controlled trial. Lumpectomy followed by radiation therapy was not associated with not reduced survival or reduced recurrence of breast cancer in the ipsilateral breast when compared to radical mastectomy and lumpectomy alone, respectively. Currently, systemic therapy is used routinely as adjuvant treatment after surgery to reduce the risk of distant micrometastases.

In-Depth [randomized controlled trial]: This trial followed 1851 women diagnosed with invasive breast tumors with positive or negative axillary lymph nodes (i.e., stage I or II). Participants were randomized to treatment total mastectomy, lumpectomy or lumpectomy followed by breast irradiation. These findings were reported after 20 years of follow-up. Breast irradiation was associated with reduced recurrence in the ipsilateral breast in women treated with lumpectomy and who had tumor-free margins on surgical specimens. The benefit of radiation therapy was independent of nodal status. At 20-year follow-up after surgery, 14.3% of women who underwent lumpectomy with radiation had a recurrence in the ipsilateral breast compared to 39.2% in women who underwent lumpectomy alone ($p < 0.001$). No significant difference was found in disease-free survival or overall survival among the 3 treatment groups.

Fisher B, Anderson S, Bryant J, Margolese RG, Deutsch M, Fisher ER, et al. Twenty-Year Follow-up of a Randomized Trial Comparing Total Mastectomy, Lumpectomy, and Lumpectomy plus Irradiation for the Treatment of Invasive Breast Cancer. The New England Journal of Medicine. 2002 Oct 17;347(16):1233–41.

The ATLAS trial: Duration of adjuvant tamoxifen in estrogen receptor-positive breast cancer

1. Among women with early estrogen receptor (ER)-positive breast cancer, continuing adjuvant tamoxifen for 10 years significantly reduced breast cancer recurrence, breast cancer mortality, and overall mortality when compared with stopping at 5 years after diagnosis.

2. Patients treated with adjuvant tamoxifen for 10 years had a significantly higher risk of endometrial cancer and pulmonary embolism

Original Date of Publication: March 2013

Study Rundown: In women with ER-positive breast cancer, previous trials had demonstrated that treatment with adjuvant tamoxifen for 5 years significantly reduced the risk of recurrence both during the treatment time and for 10 years after. During this 15-year period, mortality from breast cancer was also significantly reduced. Tamoxifen treatment, however, is linked with significantly increased risk of certain side effects, including endometrial cancer and thromboembolic disease. The Adjuvant Tamoxifen: Longer Against Shorter (ATLAS) trial compared the effects of 10 years of adjuvant tamoxifen treatment with 5 years of adjuvant tamoxifen treatment on outcomes in patients with ER-positive breast cancer. Over the duration of follow up, 10-year treatment significantly reduced breast cancer recurrence, breast cancer mortality, and overall mortality compared to the standard 5-year course of tamoxifen. However, this increased benefit came at the expense of significantly increased rates of endometrial cancer and pulmonary embolism. The study remains ongoing and future data will help elucidate the longer-term effects of prolonged tamoxifen treatment in patients with early ER-positive breast cancer.

In-Depth [randomized controlled trial]: This multinational study included 12 894 women with early breast cancer, 6454 of whom were randomized to continue tamoxifen for 10 years (i.e., the intervention group) after diagnosis and 6440 of whom were randomized to stop tamoxifen use at 5 years (i.e., the control group). While all 12 894 were included in the analysis for side effects, only women with ER-positive disease were included in the main analysis for breast cancer recurrence and mortality - 6846 women. Patients were eligible for inclusion if they had early breast cancer (i.e., completely resectable disease), they had subsequently received tamoxifen and were still on it (or had stopped in the past year and could resume treatment quickly), they were clinically free of disease (i.e., local recurrence resected, no distant recurrence), follow-up was practicable, and there was uncertainty between the patient and her physician regarding whether to continue tamoxifen treatment. There were no restrictions based on patient age, the type of initial surgery or histology, hormone receptor status, nodal status, or other treatments. Patients were not eligible if they had any contraindications to continuing tamoxifen (e.g., pregnancy, breastfeeding, retinopathy, endometrial hyperplasia).

In women with ER-positive disease, continuing tamoxifen treatment for 10 years significantly reduced the risk of breast cancer recurrence (RR 0.84; 95%CI 0.76-0.94), breast cancer mortality (RR 0.83; 95%CI 0.72-0.96), and overall mortality (RR 0.87; 95%CI 0.78-0.97) when compared to 5 years of treatment. Notably, during years 5-14 after diagnosis, the absolute recurrence reduction was 3.7% with extended tamoxifen treatment (21.4% versus 25.1%). The relative risk of pulmonary embolus (RR 1.87; 95%CI 1.13-3.07) and endometrial cancer (RR 1.74; 95%CI 1.30-2.34) were significantly higher in women who continued tamoxifen compared to the control group, while the risk of ischemic heart disease was significantly reduced (RR 0.76; 95%CI 0.60-0.95).

Davies C, Pan H, Godwin J, Gray R, Arriagada R, Raina V, et al. Long-term effects of continuing adjuvant tamoxifen to 10 years versus stopping at 5 years after diagnosis of oestrogen receptor-positive breast cancer: ATLAS, a randomised trial. Lancet. 2013 Mar 9;381(9869):805–16.

The NASCET: Carotid endarterectomy in symptomatic stenosis

1. Carotid endarterectomy, in addition to medical therapy, significantly reduced the risk of major and fatal stroke in patients with symptomatic, high-grade (70-99%) carotid stenosis.

Original Date of Publication: August 1991

Study Rundown: The North American Symptomatic Carotid Endarterectomy Trial (NASCET) was one of the first trials to provide strong evidence in favor of carotid endarterectomy, in addition to medical therapy, in treating symptomatic carotid artery stenosis. The trial was originally conceived in response to the rising rates of carotid endarterectomy without strong evidence to support its use in prophylaxis against cerebrovascular events. Results demonstrated significant benefits for patients suffering from high-grade carotid stenosis (70-99%), who had recently experienced transient ischemic attack, monocular blindness, or non-disabling stroke. These findings were consistent with findings from the European Carotid Stenosis Trial. At the time, questions remained regarding the benefits of carotid endarterectomy in patients with asymptomatic carotid stenosis, and this has been explored in subsequent trials. In summary, carotid endarterectomy in addition to medical therapy significantly reduced the absolute risk of ipsilateral stroke and major or fatal ipsilateral stroke in patients with high-grade, symptomatic, carotid artery stenosis.

In-Depth [randomized controlled trial]: Patients were recruited from 50 centers across Canada and the United States and randomized to either medical therapy alone (i.e., antiplatelet, antihypertensive, antilipid, antidiabetic therapy, as needed), or medical therapy with carotid endarterectomy. Patients were eligible for the trial if they provided informed consent, were <80 years old, and had a cerebrovascular event (i.e., transient ischemic attack, monocular blindness, non-disabling stroke) in the previous 120 days with ipsilateral carotid stenosis of 30-99% (as per carotid ultrasonography). Patients were assessed at 30 days, every three months for the first year, and every four months subsequently for death or stroke. The trial was stopped prematurely by the monitoring and executive committees according to a pre-planned rule because of evidence demonstrating treatment efficacy in patients with high-grade stenosis (70-99%) undergoing endarterectomy. The trial involving medium-grade stenosis (30-69%) continued. A total of 659 patients with high-grade stenosis were part of the final analyses. At two years, there was a significant reduction in the absolute risk of ipsilateral stroke by 17% (±3.5%, $p < 0.001$) and major or fatal ipsilateral stroke by 10.6% (±2.6%, $p < 0.001$).

North American Symptomatic Carotid Endarterectomy Trial Collaborators. Beneficial effect of carotid endarterectomy in symptomatic patients with high-grade carotid stenosis. The New England Journal of Medicine. 1991 Aug 15;325(7):445–53.

The NINDS trial: Tissue plasminogen activator in acute ischemic stroke improves functional outcomes

1. Treatment of acute ischemic stroke with tissue plasminogen activator (t-PA) within 3 hours of symptom onset significantly improved functional outcomes 3 months after stroke, when compared with placebo.

2. Tissue plasminogen activator significantly increased the rate of symptomatic intracerebral hemorrhage.

Original Date of Publication: December 1995

Study Rundown: Prior to the National Institute of Neurologic Disorders and Stroke (NINDS) trial, evidence that thrombolytic therapy benefitted patients with ischemic stroke existed, though intracerebral hemorrhage was a frequent complication. Several previous studies found that early treatment (i.e., thrombolytics within 3 hours of symptom onset) was associated with the greatest likelihood of recovery and lower risks of hemorrhage. The NINDS trial was a larger randomized controlled trial that sought to assess the efficacy of using t-PA in treating ischemic stroke within 3 hours of symptom onset. Results showed that the administration of t-PA within 3 hours of symptom onset in patients suffering ischemic stroke significantly improved functional outcomes, as observed at the 3-month mark. Patients treated with t-PA, however, suffered significantly higher rates of symptomatic bleeding. The NINDS trial was the first randomized controlled trial demonstrating that t-PA was beneficial in patients suffering from acute ischemic stroke. While the study used carefully selected sample of stroke cases, the findings of the NINDS trial formed as the basis for approving the use of thrombolytics in the management of acute strokes. It also informed the development of practice guidelines in centers across North America.

In-Depth [randomized controlled trial]: The trial consisted of 2 phases: 1) assessing for improvements in neurologic functioning within 24 hours of symptom onset to measure t-PA activity and 2) assessing for sustained clinical improvement at 3 months. In phase 1, there was no significant difference between the groups in terms of neurologic improvement within the first 24 hours. In phase 2, patients treated with t-PA demonstrated significant improvements on several functional assessment scales (i.e., NIHSS, Barthel, Modified Rankin, Glasgow Outcome) 3 months after the onset of stroke, when compared with patients in the placebo group. There were significantly more symptomatic intracerebral hemorrhages in the t-PA group, though the rate of asymptomatic intracerebral hemorrhages was not different.

The National Institute of Neurological Disorders and Stroke rt-PA Stroke Study Group. Tissue Plasminogen Activator for Acute Ischemic Stroke. The New England Journal of Medicine. 1995 Dec 14;333(24):1581–8.

The ECASS III trial: Administering alteplase up to 4.5 hours after onset of acute ischemic stroke improves neurological outcomes

1. Alteplase administered between 3 to 4.5 hours after the onset of acute ischemic stroke was associated with improved functional outcomes at 90 days, compared to placebo.

Original Date of Publication: September 2008

Study Rundown: Previously, the National Institute of Neurological Disorders and Stroke (NINDS) trial demonstrated that, compared to placebo, treatment of acute ischemic stroke with tissue plasminogen activator (t-PA) within 3 hours of symptom onset significantly improved functional outcomes 3 months after the incident. However, there remained uncertainty regarding the efficacy and safety of administering t-PA more than 3 hours after the onset of acute ischemic stroke. Two previous European trials (i.e., ECASS I and II) had investigated the use of alteplase up to 6 hours after the onset of stroke, but these studies did not demonstrate any benefits. The ECASS III trial was a randomized, controlled trial designed to explore the efficacy and safety of utilizing alteplase, a recombinant t-PA, 3 to 4.5 hours after the onset of stroke.

Treating acute ischemic stroke patients with intravenous alteplase 3 to 4.5 hours after the onset of symptoms significantly improved neurological outcomes at 3 months compared to placebo. While patients in the alteplase group experienced a significantly higher risk of intracranial hemorrhage, mortality was not significantly different between the groups. Some clinicians criticized the trial for excluding patients with severe stroke signs and for a change of protocol during the trial. Regardless, its findings have informed practice as current recommendations suggest administering recombinant t-PA up to 4.5 hours after the onset of acute ischemic stroke.

In-Depth [randomized controlled trial]: This double-blind, placebo-controlled trial examined the use of alteplase at a dose of 0.9 mg/kg. Patients were eligible for the trial if they had a stroke with a clearly defined time of onset, a measurable deficit, and a computed tomographic scan of the brain that demonstrated no evidence of intracranial hemorrhage at baseline. Exclusion criteria included stroke or serious head trauma in the preceding 3 months, major surgery in the past 14 days, history of intracranial hemorrhage, rapidly improving or minor symptoms, and seizure at the onset of stroke. The study involved 821 patients and had a primary outcome measure of disability at 90 days, as assessed using the modified Rankin Scale. The secondary outcome measure was a global measure at 90 days as determined using the modified Rankin Scale, Barthel Index, NIHSS, and Glasgow Outcome Scale. Safety outcomes included mortality at 90 days, intracranial hemorrhage (any, symptomatic), symptomatic edema, or other events. Patients in the alteplase group were significantly more likely to have favorable outcomes of both the primary and secondary outcomes when compared to the placebo group. Patients in the alteplase group, however, experienced a significantly higher risk of intracranial hemorrhage, including symptomatic intracranial hemorrhage, in the first 36 hours after treatment ($p < 0.001$). There were no significant differences between the groups in terms of mortality.

Hacke W, Kaste M, Bluhmki E, Brozman M, Dávalos A, Guidetti D, et al. Thrombolysis with Alteplase 3 to 4.5 Hours after Acute Ischemic Stroke. The New England Journal of Medicine. 2008 Sep 25;359(13):1317–29.

Initial trial of conservative management for splenic injury

1. The conservative, symptomatic management of 16 patients following assumed splenic injury from blunt abdominal trauma resulted in normalization of hemodynamic stability within 2 days of hospital admission. Furthermore, this strategy resulted in complete normalization of clinical examination by 2 weeks post-discharge, and no hospital readmissions.

2. This approach to splenic injury management was supported by subsequent investigations, eventually leading to the acceptance of conservative management as standard of care.

Original Date of Publication: October 1971

Study Rundown: The spleen is particularly susceptible to blunt abdominal trauma and, prior to this study, splenectomy was routine following abdominal injury. However, previous anecdotal evidence of the authors linked nonoperative management to positive outcomes. With the potential for spleen salvage and a reduction in surgical and post-operative risks, this study investigated the outcomes of children who were not treated surgically for their splenic injuries. The small sample size, lack of a control group, and use of descriptive statistics as the only method for analysis limited the study. In addition, conclusions drawn from the study may be inaccurate as patients were assumed to have splenic injury from clinical examination as no method, apart from surgical exploration, could confirm injury.

At the time of its publication, the proposed conservative treatment investigated in the study differed radically from expected surgical intervention. In the present day, conservative management is the preferred method of management for children with splenic injury secondary to blunt trauma. Improved imaging techniques and technology for monitoring patient hemodynamic status now allow for better assessment of the need for surgical intervention. A recent retrospective study of the evolution of splenic injury management found hospital length of stay, transfusion requirements, and mortality decreased as conservative management of splenic injury became widely accepted.

In-Depth [case-series study]: A total of 32 children admitted to the hospital during 1948-1955 following blunt abdominal trauma with potential splenic involvement were included. Six patients underwent splenectomy, 1 patient died from a crush injury, and the remaining 25 underwent nonoperative management. Of these patients, 16 were included in the study (mean age = 10 years, 69% male) as their presentation indicated likely splenic involvement, although this was not confirmed by surgical intervention. Patients underwent standard examinations with researchers reporting close monitoring of patient vitals.

All patients were conscious upon presentation with a complaint of abdominal pain and all had significant abdominal tenderness. Three children had ecchymoses overlying the site of trauma and 3 had potential intraperitoneal fluid detected on physical exam. Patient pulses ranged from 100-140/min and 4 patients had blood pressures <90/50 mmHg. Complete blood counts included hemoglobin values ranging from 7.9-11.4 g/100 mL (mean=9.5 g/100 mL) and white blood cell counts ranging from 8000-27 000 mm^3 (mean=17 000 mm^3). Patient temperatures ranged from 100°F-104°F (mean=102°F). 9 children received whole blood transfusions for hemodynamic instability and 2 received plasma. All patients received intravenous fluids. Patients were hemodynamically stable within 2 days of admission. Resolution of abdominal tenderness correlated with normalization of heart rate and body temperature. Total length of stay ranged from 4 to 42 days (mean=16 days). Two weeks after discharge, all patients' physical examinations normalized and no patient underwent readmission.

Douglas GJ, Simpson JS. The conservative management of splenic trauma. Journal of Pediatric Surgery. 1971 Oct 1;6(5):565–70.

Davies DA, Pearl RH, Ein SH, Langer JC, Wales PW. Management of blunt splenic injury in children: evolution of the nonoperative approach. Journal of Pediatric Surgery. 2009 May 1;44(5):1005–8.

The Child-Pugh score: Prognosis in chronic liver disease and cirrhosis

1. The Child-Pugh score was developed in 1973 to predict surgical outcomes in patients presenting with bleeding esophageal varices.

3. Presently, the score is used with the Model for End-Stage Liver Disease (MELD) to determine priority for liver transplantation.

Original Date of Publication: August 1973

Study Rundown: Originally developed in 1973, the Child-Pugh score estimated the risk of operative mortality in patients with bleeding esophageal varices. It has since been modified, refined, and become a widely used tool to assess prognosis in patients with chronic liver disease and cirrhosis. The score considers 5 factors, 3 of which assess the synthetic function of the liver (i.e., total bilirubin level, serum albumin, and international normalized ratio, or INR) and 2 of which are based on clinical assessment (i.e., degree of ascites and degree of hepatic encephalopathy). Critics of the Child-Pugh score have noted its reliance on clinical assessment, which may result in inconsistency in scoring. Others have suggested that its broad classifications of disease are impractical when determining priority for liver transplantation; nevertheless, it remains widely used. The MELD is a newer scoring system that has been developed to address some of the concerns with the Child-Pugh score, and both systems are often used in conjunction to determine liver transplantation priority.

In-Depth [case series study]: Thirty-eight consecutive cases of bleeding esophageal varices requiring surgery were included in the study. The severity of liver disease was assessed in each patient based on five clinical features: 1) total bilirubin level, 2) serum albumin, 3) prothrombin time (now measured as the INR), 4) the degree of ascites, and 5) the grade of hepatic encephalopathy. The total point score was used to determine the patient's Child-Pugh class (Table I.). Class A patients (n=7) experienced a 29% operative mortality rate, while Class B (n=13) and Class C (n=18) patients had operative mortality rates of 38% and 88%, respectively. Since its publication, the Child-Pugh score has undergone modifications and is currently used to assess the severity and prognosis of chronic liver disease and cirrhosis. It is often used together with the MELD to determine the priority for liver transplantation. The current Child-Pugh scoring system is outlined below.

Pugh RNH, Murray-Lyon IM, Dawson JL, Pietroni MC, Williams R. Transection of the oesophagus for bleeding oesophageal varices. Br J Surg. 1973 Aug 1;60(8):646–9.

Child-Pugh Score			
Factor	**1 point**	**2 points**	**3 points**
Total bilirubin (μmol/L)	<34	34-50	>50
Serum albumin (g/L)	>35	28-35	<28
PT INR	<1.7	1.71-2.30	>2.30
Ascites	None	Mild	Moderate to Severe
Hepatic encephalopathy	None	Grade I-II (or suppressed with medication)	Grade III-IV (or refractory)

	Class A	**Class B**	**Class C**
Total points	5-6	7-9	10-15
1-year survival	100%	80%	45%

Table I. Child-Pugh score.

The Harvey-Bradshaw Index is a practical alternative to the Crohn's Disease Activity Index in measuring disease severity

1. The Crohn's Disease Activity Index (CDAI) is accurate in quantifying disease severity in patients with Crohn's disease, but is cumbersome in practice.

2. The Harvey-Bradshaw Index (HBI) is a practical alternative that is simpler and has been statistically validated.

Original Date of Publication: March 1980

Study Rundown: Crohn's disease in a disorder of unidentified etiology characterized by inflammation of the gastrointestinal tract. The course tends to follow a chronic pattern of remissions and exacerbations with significant variability of organ distribution, yielding a broad spectrum of clinical presentations. The CDAI was developed as a research tool in an attempt to quantify the degree of illness. It gives a score based on a diary of symptoms kept by the patient for 7 days, taking into account other measurements such as the patient's weight and hematocrit. While the CDAI has been shown to be accurate in assessing disease severity and avoiding a single 'good or bad day' bias, it is criticized as too burdensome for routine practice.

The HBI was devised as a simpler version of the CDAI. It consists of only clinical parameters, does not require biochemical tests, and is far simpler to use than the CDAI. Best, a contributor to the CDAI, drew statistically significant correlations between the HBI and CDAI using prediction limits. Vermeire et al. further validated these correlations using statistical analysis of 2 large multicenter prospective cohort studies (PEGylated antibody fragment evaluation in Crohn's disease: safety and efficacy – PRECiSE 1 and 2). Both indicated that the HBI is a good – though imperfect – substitute for the CDAI in evaluating disease severity. These results support the use of the HBI for routine practice, reserving the CDAI for clinical trials requiring high accuracy.

In-Depth [prospective cohort]: The CDAI is based on 8 parameters, each adjusted using a weighting factor (indicated in parentheses), as follows: number of liquid or soft stools each day for seven days (x2), abdominal pain each day for seven days (x5), general well-being each day for seven days (x7), presence of complications (x20), taking Lomotil or opiates to control diarrhea (x30), presence of an abdominal mass (x10), hematocrit of under 0.47 in men and 0.42 in women (x6), and percentage deviation from standard weight (x1). Points are added for clinical findings of arthritis, uveitis, fistulae or abscesses, fevers, and other complications. Remission of disease is defined as a score below 150 and severe disease is defined as a value greater than 450. The HBI uses only 5 items: general well-being, abdominal pain, number of liquid stools per day, abdominal mass, and complications. The first three of these are scored from the previous day to reduce bias.

112 patients attending a gastroenterology clinic were assessed with both the CDAI and the HBI on the same visit. The results were then plotted and regression analysis was run to assess the correlation between the two methods of data collection. The results indicated a positive correlation of 0.93 ($p < 0.001$). The results of PRECiSE 1 and 2 indicated a pooled correlation of 0.800 (0.780 – 0.819 confidence interval). This is in close agreement with Best's finding of a 27-point change in the CDAI for every point change in the HBI.

Harvey RF, Bradshaw JM. A Simple Index of Crohn's-Disease Activity. The Lancet. 1980 Mar 8;315(8167):514.

Additional Review:

Vermeire S, Schreiber S, Sandborn WJ, Dubois C, Rutgeerts P. Correlation between the Crohn's disease activity and Harvey–Bradshaw indices in assessing Crohn's disease severity. Clinical Gastroenterology and Hepatology. 2010 Apr 30;8(4):357-63.

Best WR. Predicting the Crohn's disease activity index from the Harvey-Bradshaw index. Inflammatory bowel diseases. 2006 Apr 1;12(4):304-10.

Harvey-Bradshaw Index	
Symptom	**Severity score**
General well-being	0 = very well 1 = slightly below par 2 = poor 3 = very poor 4 = terrible
Abdominal pain	0 = none 1 = mild 2 = moderate 3 = severe
Number of liquid stools daily	1 per occurrence
Abdominal mass	0 = none 1 = dubious 2 = definite 3 = definite and tender
Complications	1 per item: – Arthralgia – Uveitis – Erythema nodosum – Aphthous ulcer – Pyoderma gangrenosum – Anal fissure – New fistula – Abscess

Table I. Harvey-Bradshaw Index. The index is based on five variables that are added to give a total score. Evaluation is done over a single day. General well-being, abdominal pain, and number of liquid stools daily are in based on the previous day.

Crohn's Disease Activity Index		
Variable	**Scale**	**Weight**
Liquid or very soft stool	Daily stool count summed for 7 days	2
Abdominal pain	Sum of 7 days of daily ratings as: 0=none 1=mild 2=moderate 3=severe	5
General well-being	Sum of 7 days of daily ratings as: 0=generally well 1=slightly below par 2=poor 3=very poor 4=terrible	7
Features of extraintestinal disease	Presence of any of the following in the previous 7 days: – Arthritis or arthralgia – Skin or mouth lesions – Iritis or uveitis – Anal fissures, fistulas, perianal abscess – Other external fistulas – Fever >100°F	20 each
Opiates for diarrhea	0=no 1=yes	30
Abdominal mass	0=none 2=questionable 5=definite	10
Hematocrit	Men 47% hematocrit Women 42% hematocrit	6
Body weight	100 x [1-(body weight/standard weight)]	1

Table II. Crohn's Disease Activity Index. Compared to the HBI, three additional variables are evaluated (opiate use, hematocrit, and body weight). Each variable is given a relative weight. the index also is tracked over a week-long period.

The Milan Criteria: Liver transplantation is effective for treating cirrhotic patients with unrespectable hepatocellular carcinoma

1. Patients with cirrhosis and unresectable hepatocellular carcinoma (HCC), either 1 tumor less than 5 cm or no more than 3 tumors less than 3 cm (Milan Criteria), who received orthotopic liver transplants (OLTs) had a 75% 4-year actuarial survival rate and an 83% rate of recurrence-free survival.

2. Patients who's excised livers showed their HCCs were accurately staged and met Milan Criteria had statistically better survival rates than patients whose tumors where mistakenly staged too low and included in the study.

Original Date of Publication: March 1996

Study Rundown: HCC is a primary liver malignancy that often occurs in patients with chronic liver disease and cirrhosis. The development of cirrhosis and subsequent HCC is closely associated with liver damage by causes such as chronic hepatitis infections, alcohol abuse, or genetic causes. Symptoms of advanced HCC include upper right quadrant abdominal pain, an enlarged abdomen, and weight loss. Screening of known cirrhotic patients using imaging or the alpha-fetoprotein (AFP) blood biomarker now allows many HCCs to be diagnosed early. Prognosis for patients with HCC has been poor, with 5-year survival rates ranging from approx. 20-40%.

Retrospective studies have suggested OLT may be a beneficial treatment compared to liver resection, especially for early stage HCC. In this small study of 48 patients with unrespectable, early stage HCC as defined by the size and number of tumors present were given orthotopic liver transplants and followed up to assess survival and recurrence. Results showed patients meeting the criteria of the study as verified by pathological examination of the liver had a significantly better 4-year survival and recurrence outcomes than patients with more advanced cancers. The Milan criteria established in this study indicating

OLT for early-stage HCC has good prognosis has been used in policy by insurers and organ networks to help select patients most likely to benefit from the procedure. A larger prospective cohort by Duffy and colleagues indicated that HCC at a later stage, defined by the UCSF criteria as 1 tumor less than 6.5 cm in diameter, a maximum of 3 total tumors with none greater than 4.5 cm in diameter, and cumulative tumor size less than 8 cm, did not have statistically different 5-year post transplant survival rates.

In-Depth [prospective cohort]: This prospective trial was conducted at The National Cancer Institute in Milan, Italy. Patients with unresectable HCC due to multifocality, inoperable location, or causing hepatic insufficiency were evaluated for inclusion in this study (n=295). Histologic confirmation of cirrhosis and histologic or serum confirmation of early stage HCC deemed 60 patients eligible for the study. Eligible patients were assessed via hepatic angiography and liver CT scans to confirm there was 1 tumor less than 5 cm in diameter or no more than 3 tumors each less than 3 cm in diameter. Suspicion or evidence of tumor invasion into blood vessels or lymph nodes excluded patients from the study. The study followed 48 patients (38 male, median age 52, age range 39-60) who met these criteria. Cirrhosis was caused by hepatitis infection in 45 patients. Liver function was assessed using Child-Pugh classification. Most patients classified as having intermediate or poor hepatic function (Child-Pugh class A or B) received anticancer treatment prior to transplantation (n=26). All patients with normal liver function (n=15) and some with intermediate or poor function (n=5) were not pretreated with anticancer regimens. Liver transplantations were performed when a compatible liver became available. Tumor stage follow-up using ultrasound, chest radiography, and serum AFP was performed every 3 months after transplantation, abdominal and chest CT scans were performed every 6 months, and radionuclide bone scans were performed every 8 months.

Follow-up time for patients in this study was a median of 26 months (range 9-54). Death following transplantation occurred in 8 patients, and 2 patients required retransplantation due to recurrent viral hepatitis. Cancer recurrence occurred in 4 patients at a median of 4 months following transplantation. For all patients who underwent liver transplantation, the survival rate at 4 years was 75% and recurrence-free survival was 83%. Survival was statistically not affected by patient age, sex, preoperative anticancer treatment, or common markers of chronic liver disease (T stage, number of tumors, serum AFP levels, and presence of a capsule). Pathological examination of excised livers indicated 13 patients (27%) had tumors that did not meet the study criteria regarding size/number of tumors. For patients who were preoperatively staged accurately, the 4-year overall survival rate was 85% and recurrence freed survival rate was 92%. Those mistakenly understaged had 4-year overall and recurrence free survival rates of 50 and 59%, respectively.

Mazzaferro V, Regalia E, Doci R, Andreola S, Pulvirenti A, Bozzetti F, et al. Liver Transplantation for the Treatment of Small Hepatocellular Carcinomas in Patients with Cirrhosis. New England Journal of Medicine. 1996 Mar 14;334(11):693–700.

Additional Review:

Duffy JP, Vardanian A, Benjamin E, Watson M, Farmer DG, Ghobrial RM, et al. Liver Transplantation Criteria For Hepatocellular Carcinoma Should Be Expanded. Ann Surg. 2007 Sep;246(3):502–11.

The MELD score: Predicting survival in end-stage liver disease

1. The Model for End-Stage Liver Disease (MELD) is a reliable tool for predicting short-term survival in patients with advanced liver disease.

2. The score is generalizable to diverse etiologies and a wide range of disease severity.

Original Date of Publication: February 2001

Study Rundown: The MELD was originally developed to predict outcomes in patients after a transjugular intrahepatic portosystemic shunt (TIPS) procedure. This study assessed whether the model could reliably predict short-term survival in patients with chronic liver disease. The investigators found that MELD scores were a good predictor of 1-week, 3-month and 1-year survival, which had important implications for the model's use in the allocation of donor livers. Previously, the Child-Turcotte-Pugh (CTP) system was used to rank patients according to urgency and medical need, however the broad classifications made it difficult to rank patients according to severity of disease. Another issue with CTP scores was the subjectivity involved in some of the criteria (e.g., assessment of ascites and encephalopathy). The MELD criteria were an improvement on these aspects of CTP scores as patients were assigned a numerical score based on objective measures.

In-Depth [cohort study]: This study evaluated the validity of the MELD score for predicting survival in patients with end-stage liver disease. The model used measures of serum creatinine, total serum bilirubin, International Normalized Ratio (INR) for prothrombin time and etiology of cirrhosis to assess disease severity. The model was assessed in 4 independent samples, which included patients hospitalized with advanced end-stage liver disease, ambulatory patients with noncholestatic cirrhosis, ambulatory patients with primary biliary cirrhosis (PBC) and a historical group of cirrhotic patients from a period when liver transplantation was not widely available. The primary outcome measure was 3-month survival and validity was also assessed for predicting 1-week and 1-year survival. The C statistics for 3-month mortality in the hospitalized, ambulatory noncholestatic, ambulatory PBC and historical groups respectively were 0.87, 0.80, 0.87 and 0.78. These values changed minimally when etiology of disease was excluded from the model. The MELD score was found to be a reliable tool to predict survival in patients with chronic liver disease.

Kamath PS, Wiesner RH, Malinchoc M, Kremers W, Therneau TM, Kosberg CL, et al. A model to predict survival in patients with end-stage liver disease. Hepatology. 2001 Feb 1;33(2):464–70.

Intraperitoneal chemotherapy improves advanced ovarian cancer survival

1. Women with advanced-stage (≥Stage III) ovarian cancer randomized to intraperitoneal chemotherapy achieved an increase in overall survival compared to controls.

Original Date of Publication: January 2006

Study Rundown: Ovarian cancer is the deadliest gynecologic malignancy. Due to nonspecific presenting symptoms and disease predilection for early intraabdominal spread via peritoneal lymphatics, the majority of patients present with advanced-stage disease. As of the early 2000s, the standard of care for women with advanced disease involved optimal tumor reductive surgery, defined as resection of all disease >1 cm, followed by adjuvant intravenous chemotherapy. The most common chemotherapy regimen involved 6 cycles of paclitaxel and a platinum analogue, such as cisplatin. The peritoneal cavity is the primary site of disease in ovarian cancer, which triggered researchers to postulate that applying chemotherapy locally to the peritoneal cavity might improve disease response and decrease toxicities associated with intravenous chemotherapy. Previous trials comparing intravenous only (IV) versus intravenous plus intraperitoneal (IV/IP) chemotherapy produced mixed results: one demonstrated a significant survival advantage in the IV/IP group while another showed an improvement in the progression-free interval but not survival.

This landmark Phase 3 clinical trial compared the standard of care, IV cisplatin/paclitaxel, to IV paclitaxel with IP cisplatin/paclitaxel and found that the IV/IP regimen was associated with increase in both progression-free survival and overall survival. However, the minority (<50%) of patients in the IV/IP group completed 6 cycles of treatment due to toxicities including fatigue, pain and neurologic side effects. Findings changed clinical practice such that patients with advanced-stage ovarian cancer who seek to maximize survival at the cost of an increased risk of treatment-associated toxicities are now offered IP chemotherapy. Strengths included parsimonious, multicenter, randomized controlled trial through the Gynecologic Oncology Group (GOG). Central review of the complete medical record by GOG physician-scientists permitted adherence to strict inclusion and exclusion criteria. Findings are limited by a low completion rate of IV/IP regimen due to toxicities, which may bias results toward the null.

In-Depth [randomized controlled trial]: A total of 415 women with Stage III ovarian carcinoma or primary peritoneal carcinoma who underwent optimal tumor reductive surgery (no residual mass greater than 1.0 cm) were randomized to receive intravenous cisplatin/paclitaxel ("IV," n=210) or intravenous paclitaxel followed by intraperitoneal cisplatin/paclitaxel ("IV/IP," n=205) for 6 cycles of chemotherapy occurring every three weeks at one of the Gynecologic Oncology Group (GOG) clinical centers across the United States (Columbus, New York, Irvine, Philadelphia, Oklahoma, Baltimore). Primary outcome was duration of overall survival. Secondary outcomes included progression-free survival, quality of life and treatment-associated toxicities.

Among women with Stage III ovarian cancer who underwent optimal tumor reductive surgery, those randomized to IV/IP chemotherapy experienced an increased duration of overall survival (67 versus 50 months, $p = 0.03$) and a longer progression-free survival (24 versus 18 months, $p = 0.05$) compared to those randomized to IV chemotherapy. Compared to women receiving standard IV chemotherapy alone, women in the IV/IP group were more likely to report toxicities including fatigue, pain and neurologic side effects but experienced a similar quality of life 1 year after treatment.

Armstrong DK, Bundy B, Wenzel L, Huang HQ, Baergen R, Lele S, et al. Intraperitoneal cisplatin and paclitaxel in ovarian cancer. The New England Journal of Medicine. 2006;354(1):34-43.

The PIVOT: Radical prostatectomy versus observation

1. Prostatectomy did not significantly reduce all-cause mortality or prostate cancer mortality when compared to observation.

2. These findings supported conservative management for men with localized prostate cancer, especially for those with prostate-specific antigen (PSA) values less than 10 ng/mL and low-risk disease.

Original Date of Publication: July 2012

Study Rundown: The incidence of prostate cancer in men is relatively high, but high long-term survival rates have been observed with conservative management. The treatment of localized prostate cancer is controversial, as few trials have compared surgical intervention to observation in the time since PSA testing has become a common screening tool. The Prostate Cancer Intervention versus Observation Trial (PIVOT) found no significant difference in all-cause or prostate-cancer mortality following radical prostatectomy compared to observation. These findings suggest that observation is a safe strategy in managing localized prostate cancer and avoids the unnecessary risks of intervention. The results also showed that PSA levels and tumor risk may be useful in identifying patients who will benefit from radical prostatectomy. Strengths of the study include the representative sample and measurement of all-cause mortality as the primary outcome, which avoids biased assessments of cause-of-death. Of note, the study may have been underpowered as the investigators intended to enroll 2000 participants, but reduced the sample size to 731. In addition, a substantial number of patients did not adhere to the assigned treatment in both groups, which could influence the observed treatment effect.

In-Depth [randomized controlled trial]: The trial included 731 men and followed participants for a median of 10 years. Patients were recruited from 44 Department of Veteran Affairs sites and 8 National Cancer Institute sites. In order to be eligible for the trial, patients had to be fit for radical prostatectomy, have histologically confirmed, clinically localized prostate cancer of any grade diagnosed within the previous 12 months, have PSA <50 ng/mL, be ≤75 years of age, a negative bone scan, and life expectancy of at least 10 years from randomization. The primary outcome was all-cause mortality and a secondary outcome was prostate-cancer mortality, defined as death due to prostate cancer or prostate cancer treatment. The rate of all-cause mortality was not significantly different between the two groups (HR 0.88; 95%CI 0.71-1.08). There was also no significant difference between groups in prostate cancer mortality (HR 0.63; 95%CI 0.36-1.09). A significant interaction was found between study group and baseline PSA value. In men with a PSA value greater than 10 ng/mL, a significant reduction in all-cause mortality was observed with surgery ($p = 0.04$), though surgery did not reduce all-cause mortality in men with a PSA less than or equal to 10 ng/mL.

Wilt TJ, Brawer MK, Jones KM, Barry MJ, Aronson WJ, Fox S, et al. Radical Prostatectomy versus Observation for Localized Prostate Cancer. The New England Journal of Medicine. 2012 Jul 19;367(3):203–13.

Index

Bibliography

This bibliography includes any references, such as original trials and follow-up trials, in this text. References are in descending order by publication date.

1. PI-RADS [Internet]. 2018 [cited 2018 Dec 7]. Available from: https://www.acr.org/Clinical-Resources/Reporting-and-Data-Systems/PI-RADS

2. Lung Rads [Internet]. 2018 [cited 2018 Dec 7]. Available from: https://www.acr.org/Clinical-Resources/Reporting-and-Data-Systems/Lung-Rads

3. Breast Imaging Reporting & Data System | American College of Radiology [Internet]. 2018 [cited 2018 Dec 7]. Available from: https://www.acr.org/Clinical-Resources/Reporting-and-Data-Systems/Bi-Rads

4. Nogueira RG, Jadhav AP, Haussen DC, Bonafe A, Budzik RF, Bhuva P, et al. Thrombectomy 6 to 24 Hours after Stroke with a Mismatch between Deficit and Infarct. New England Journal of Medicine. 2018 Jan 4;378(1):11–21.

5. Campbell BCV, Mitchell PJ, Churilov L, Yassi N, Kleinig TJ, Dowling RJ, et al. Tenecteplase versus Alteplase before Thrombectomy for Ischemic Stroke. New England Journal of Medicine. 2018 Apr 26;378(17):1573–82.

6. Campbell BCV, Mitchell PJ, Churilov L, Yassi N, Kleinig TJ, Dowling RJ, et al. Tenecteplase versus Alteplase before Thrombectomy for Ischemic Stroke. N Engl J Med. 2018 26;378(17):1573–82.

7. Albers GW, Marks MP, Kemp S, Christensen S, Tsai JP, Ortega-Gutierrez S, et al. Thrombectomy for Stroke at 6 to 16 Hours with Selection by Perfusion Imaging. N Engl J Med. 2018 22;378(8):708–18.

8. Sweeting MJ, Patel R, Powell JT, Greenhalgh RM, EVAR Trial Investigators. Endovascular Repair of Abdominal Aortic Aneurysm in Patients Physically Ineligible for Open Repair: Very Long-term Follow-up in the EVAR-2 Randomized Controlled Trial. Ann Surg. 2017;266(5):713–9.

9. MacMahon H, Naidich DP, Goo JM, Lee KS, Leung ANC, Mayo JR, et al. Guidelines for Management of Incidental Pulmonary Nodules Detected on CT Images: From the Fleischner Society 2017. Radiology. 2017 Feb 23;284(1):228–43.

10. Saver JL, Goyal M, Bonafe A, Diener H-C, Levy EI, Pereira VM, et al. Stent-Retriever Thrombectomy after Intravenous t-PA vs. t-PA Alone in Stroke. New England Journal of Medicine. 2015 Jun 11;372(24):2285–95.

11. Mitchell DG, Bruix J, Sherman M, Sirlin CB. LI-RADS (Liver Imaging Reporting and Data System): Summary, discussion, and consensus of the LI-RADS Management Working Group and future directions. Hepatology. 2015 Mar 1;61(3):1056–65.

12. Jovin TG, Chamorro A, Cobo E, de Miquel MA, Molina CA, Rovira A, et al. Thrombectomy within 8 Hours after Symptom Onset in Ischemic Stroke. New England Journal of Medicine. 2015 Jun 11;372(24):2296–306.

13. Goyal M, Demchuk AM, Menon BK, Eesa M, Rempel JL, Thornton J, et al. Randomized Assessment of Rapid Endovascular Treatment of Ischemic Stroke. New England Journal of Medicine. 2015 Mar 12;372(11):1019–30.

14. Douglas PS, Hoffmann U, Patel MR, Mark DB, Al-Khalidi HR, Cavanaugh B, et al. Outcomes of Anatomical versus Functional Testing for Coronary Artery Disease. New England Journal of Medicine. 2015 Apr 2;372(14):1291–300.

15. Campbell BCV, Mitchell PJ, Kleinig TJ, Dewey HM, Churilov L, Yassi N, et al. Endovascular Therapy for Ischemic Stroke with Perfusion-Imaging Selection. New England Journal of Medicine. 2015 Mar 12;372(11):1009–18.

16. Berkhemer OA, Fransen PSS, Beumer D, van den Berg LA, Lingsma HF, Yoo AJ, et al. A Randomized Trial of Intraarterial Treatment for Acute Ischemic Stroke. New England Journal of Medicine. 2015 Jan 1;372(1):11–20.

17. Friedewald SM, Rafferty EA, Rose SL, Durand MA, Plecha DM, Greenberg JS, et al. Breast Cancer Screening Using Tomosynthesis in Combination With Digital Mammography. JAMA. 2014 Jun 25;311(24):2499–507.

18. Wald C, Russo MW, Heimbach JK, Hussain HK, Pomfret EA, Bruix J. New OPTN/UNOS Policy for Liver Transplant Allocation: Standardization of Liver Imaging, Diagnosis, Classification, and Reporting of Hepatocellular Carcinoma. Radiology. 2013 Feb 1;266(2):376–82.

19. Naidich DP, Bankier AA, MacMahon H, Schaefer-Prokop CM, Pistolesi M, Goo JM, et al. Recommendations for the management of subsolid pulmonary nodules detected at CT: a statement from the Fleischner Society. Radiology. 2013 Jan;266(1):304–17.

20. Miglioretti DL, Johnson E, Williams A, Greenlee RT, Weinmann S, Solberg LI, et al. The use of computed tomography in pediatrics and the associated radiation exposure and estimated cancer risk. JAMA Pediatr. 2013 Aug 1;167(8):700–7.

21. Guérin C, Reignier J, Richard J-C, Beuret P, Gacouin A, Boulain T, et al. Prone Positioning in Severe Acute Respiratory Distress Syndrome. New England Journal of Medicine. 2013 Jun 6;368(23):2159–68.

22. Davies C, Pan H, Godwin J, Gray R, Arriagada R, Raina V, et al. Long-term effects of continuing adjuvant tamoxifen to 10 years versus stopping at 5 years after diagnosis of oestrogen receptor-positive breast cancer: ATLAS, a randomised trial. The Lancet. 2013 Mar 9;381(9869):805–16.

23. Wilt TJ, Brawer MK, Jones KM, Barry MJ, Aronson WJ, Fox S, et al. Radical Prostatectomy versus Observation for Localized Prostate Cancer. New England Journal of Medicine. 2012 Jul 19;367(3):203–13.

24. Schoen RE, Pinsky PF, Weissfeld JL, Yokochi LA, Church T, Laiyemo AO, et al. Colorectal-Cancer Incidence and Mortality with Screening Flexible Sigmoidoscopy. New England Journal of Medicine. 2012 Jun 21;366(25):2345–57.

25. Pearce MS, Salotti JA, Little MP, McHugh K, Lee C, Kim KP, et al. Radiation exposure from CT scans in childhood and subsequent risk of leukaemia and brain tumours: a retrospective cohort study. The Lancet. 2012 Aug 4;380(9840):499–505.

26. Hoffmann U, Truong QA, Schoenfeld DA, Chou ET, Woodard PK, Nagurney JT, et al. Coronary CT Angiography versus Standard Evaluation in Acute Chest Pain. New England Journal of Medicine. 2012 Jul 26;367(4):299–308.

27. National Lung Screening Trial Research Team, Aberle DR, Adams AM, Berg CD, Black WC, Clapp JD, et al. Reduced lung-cancer mortality with low-dose computed tomographic screening. N Engl J Med. 2011 Aug 4;365(5):395–409.

28. Jolly SS, Yusuf S, Cairns J, Niemelä K, Xavier D, Widimsky P, et al. Radial versus femoral access for coronary angiography and intervention in patients with acute coronary syndromes (RIVAL): a randomised, parallel group, multicentre trial. The Lancet. 2011 Apr 23;377(9775):1409–20.

29. Chimowitz MI, Lynn MJ, Derdeyn CP, Turan TN, Fiorella D, Lane BF, et al. Stenting versus aggressive medical therapy for intracranial arterial stenosis. N Engl J Med. 2011 Sep 15;365(11):993–1003.

30. Buys SS, Partridge E, Black A, Johnson CC, Lamerato L, Isaacs C, et al. Effect of Screening on Ovarian Cancer Mortality: The Prostate, Lung, Colorectal and Ovarian (PLCO) Cancer Screening Randomized Controlled Trial. JAMA. 2011 Jun 8;305(22):2295–303.

31. van Santvoort HC, Besselink MG, Bakker OJ, Hofker HS, Boermeester MA, Dejong CH, et al. A Step-up Approach or Open Necrosectomy for Necrotizing Pancreatitis. New England Journal of Medicine. 2010 Apr 22;362(16):1491–502.

32. United Kingdom EVAR Trial Investigators, Greenhalgh RM, Brown LC, Powell JT, Thompson SG, Epstein D. Endovascular repair of aortic aneurysm in patients physically ineligible for open repair. N Engl J Med. 2010 May 20;362(20):1872–80.

33. TOMA N. Endovascular versus open repair of abdominal aortic aneurysm. Maedica (Buchar). 2010 Apr;5(2):148.

34. García-Pagán JC, Caca K, Bureau C, Laleman W, Appenrodt B, Luca A, et al. Early Use of TIPS in Patients with Cirrhosis and Variceal Bleeding. New England Journal of Medicine. 2010 Jun 24;362(25):2370–9.

35. Brott TG, Hobson RW, Howard G, Roubin GS, Clark WM, Brooks W, et al. Stenting versus Endarterectomy for Treatment of Carotid-Artery Stenosis. New England Journal of Medicine. 2010 Jul 1;363(1):11–23.

36. Wolchok JD, Hoos A, O'Day S, Weber JS, Hamid O, Lebbé C, et al. Guidelines for the Evaluation of Immune Therapy Activity in Solid Tumors: Immune-Related Response Criteria. Clin Cancer Res. 2009 Dec 1;15(23):7412–20.

37. Serruys PW, Morice M-C, Kappetein AP, Colombo A, Holmes DR, Mack MJ, et al. Percutaneous Coronary Intervention versus Coronary-Artery Bypass Grafting for Severe Coronary Artery Disease. New England Journal of Medicine. 2009 Mar 5;360(10):961–72.

38. Rimola J, Rodriguez S, García-Bosch O, Ordás I, Ayala E, Aceituno M, et al. Magnetic resonance for assessment of disease activity and severity in ileocolonic Crohn's disease. Gut. 2009 Aug 1;58(8):1113–20.

39. Kuppermann N, Holmes JF, Dayan PS, Hoyle JD, Atabaki SM, Holubkov R, et al. Identification of children at very low risk of clinically-important brain injuries after head trauma: a prospective cohort study. The Lancet. 2009 Oct 3;374(9696):1160–70.

40. Kallmes DF, Comstock BA, Heagerty PJ, Turner JA, Wilson DJ, Diamond TH, et al. A Randomized Trial of Vertebroplasty for Osteoporotic Spinal Fractures. New England Journal of Medicine. 2009 Aug 6;361(6):569–79.

41. Hoffmann U, Bamberg F, Chae CU, Nichols JH, Rogers IS, Seneviratne SK, et al. Coronary Computed Tomography Angiography For Early Triage of Patients with Acute Chest Pain - The Rule Out Myocardial Infarction Using Computer Assisted Tomography (ROMICAT) Trial. J Am Coll Cardiol. 2009 May 5;53(18):1642–50.

42. González AB de, Mahesh M, Kim K-P, Bhargavan M, Lewis R, Mettler F, et al. Projected Cancer Risks From Computed Tomographic Scans Performed in the United States in 2007. Arch Intern Med. 2009 Dec 14;169(22):2071–7.

43. Eisenhauer EA, Therasse P, Bogaerts J, Schwartz LH, Sargent D, Ford R, et al. New response evaluation criteria in solid tumours: Revised RECIST guideline (version 1.1). European Journal of Cancer. 2009 Jan 1;45(2):228–47.

44. Baumann P, Nyman J, Hoyer M, Wennberg B, Gagliardi G, Lax I, et al. Outcome in a Prospective Phase II Trial of Medically Inoperable Stage I

Non–Small-Cell Lung Cancer Patients Treated With Stereotactic Body Radiotherapy. JCO. 2009 Jul 10;27(20):3290–6.

45. Andriole GL, Crawford ED, Grubb RL, Buys SS, Chia D, Church TR, et al. Mortality Results from a Randomized Prostate-Cancer Screening Trial. New England Journal of Medicine. 2009 Mar 26;360(13):1310–9.

46. Lencioni R, Crocetti L, Cioni R, Suh R, Glenn D, Regge D, et al. Response to radiofrequency ablation of pulmonary tumours: a prospective, intention-to-treat, multicentre clinical trial (the RAPTURE study). The Lancet Oncology. 2008 Jul 1;9(7):621–8.

47. Hacke W, Kaste M, Bluhmki E, Brozman M, Dávalos A, Guidetti D, et al. Thrombolysis with Alteplase 3 to 4.5 Hours after Acute Ischemic Stroke. New England Journal of Medicine. 2008 Sep 25;359(13):1317–29.

48. Kim DH, Pickhardt PJ, Taylor AJ, Leung WK, Winter TC, Hinshaw JL, et al. CT Colonography versus Colonoscopy for the Detection of Advanced Neoplasia. New England Journal of Medicine. 2007 Oct 4;357(14):1403–12.

49. Boyd NF, Guo H, Martin LJ, Sun L, Stone J, Fishell E, et al. Mammographic Density and the Risk and Detection of Breast Cancer. New England Journal of Medicine. 2007 Jan 18;356(3):227–36.

50. Boden WE, O'Rourke RA, Teo KK, Hartigan PM, Maron DJ, Kostuk WJ, et al. Optimal Medical Therapy with or without PCI for Stable Coronary Disease. New England Journal of Medicine. 2007 Apr 12;356(15):1503–16.

51. Stein PD, Fowler SE, Goodman LR, Gottschalk A, Hales CA, Hull RD, et al. Multidetector Computed Tomography for Acute Pulmonary Embolism. New England Journal of Medicine. 2006 Jun 1;354(22):2317–27.

52. Pedrosa I, Levine D, Eyvazzadeh AD, Siewert B, Ngo L, Rofsky NM. MR imaging evaluation of acute appendicitis in pregnancy. Radiology. 2006 Mar;238(3):891–9.

53. Grobner T. Gadolinium – a specific trigger for the development of nephrogenic fibrosing dermopathy and nephrogenic systemic fibrosis? Nephrol Dial Transplant. 2006 Apr 1;21(4):1104–8.

54. Armstrong DK, Bundy B, Wenzel L, Huang HQ, Baergen R, Lele S, et al. Intraperitoneal Cisplatin and Paclitaxel in Ovarian Cancer. New England Journal of Medicine. 2006 Jan 5;354(1):34–43.

55. MacMahon H, Austin JHM, Gamsu G, Herold CJ, Jett JR, Naidich DP, et al. Guidelines for Management of Small Pulmonary Nodules Detected on CT Scans: A Statement from the Fleischner Society. Radiology. 2005 Nov 1;237(2):395–400.

56. Kinkel K, Lu Y, Mehdizade A, Pelte M-F, Hricak H. Indeterminate Ovarian Mass at US: Incremental Value of Second Imaging Test for

Characterization—Meta-Analysis and Bayesian Analysis. Radiology. 2005 Jul 1;236(1):85–94.

57. de Winter RJ, Windhausen F, Cornel JH, Dunselman PHJM, Janus CL, Bendermacher PEF, et al. Early Invasive versus Selectively Invasive Management for Acute Coronary Syndromes. New England Journal of Medicine. 2005 Sep 15;353(11):1095–104.

58. McFalls EO, Ward HB, Moritz TE, Goldman S, Krupski WC, Littooy F, et al. Coronary-Artery Revascularization before Elective Major Vascular Surgery. New England Journal of Medicine. 2004 Dec 30;351(27):2795–804.

59. Kriege M, Brekelmans CTM, Boetes C, Besnard PE, Zonderland HM, Obdeijn IM, et al. Efficacy of MRI and Mammography for Breast-Cancer Screening in Women with a Familial or Genetic Predisposition. New England Journal of Medicine. 2004 Jul 29;351(5):427–37.

60. Wells PS, Anderson DR, Rodger M, Forgie M, Kearon C, Dreyer J, et al. Evaluation of D-Dimer in the Diagnosis of Suspected Deep-Vein Thrombosis. New England Journal of Medicine. 2003 Sep 25;349(13):1227–35.

61. Stiell IG, Clement CM, McKnight RD, Brison R, Schull MJ, Rowe BH, et al. The Canadian C-Spine Rule versus the NEXUS Low-Risk Criteria in Patients with Trauma. New England Journal of Medicine. 2003 Dec 25;349(26):2510–8.

62. Lencioni RA, Allgaier H-P, Cioni D, Olschewski M, Deibert P, Crocetti L, et al. Small Hepatocellular Carcinoma in Cirrhosis: Randomized Comparison of Radio-frequency Thermal Ablation versus Percutaneous Ethanol Injection. Radiology. 2003 Jul 1;228(1):235–40.

63. Gervais DA, McGovern FJ, Arellano RS, McDougal WS, Mueller PR. Renal Cell Carcinoma: Clinical Experience and Technical Success with Radio-frequency Ablation of 42 Tumors. Radiology. 2003 Feb 1;226(2):417–24.

64. Fishman A, Martinez F, Naunheim K, Piantadosi S, Wise R, Ries A, et al. A randomized trial comparing lung-volume-reduction surgery with medical therapy for severe emphysema. N Engl J Med. 2003 May 22;348(21):2059–73.

65. Molyneux A. International Subarachnoid Aneurysm Trial (ISAT) of neurosurgical clipping versus endovascular coiling in 2143 patients with ruptured intracranial aneurysms: a randomised trial. The Lancet. 2002 Oct 26;360(9342):1267–74.

66. Llovet JM, Real MI, Montaña X, Planas R, Coll S, Aponte J, et al. Arterial embolisation or chemoembolisation versus symptomatic treatment in patients with unresectable hepatocellular carcinoma: a randomised controlled trial. The Lancet. 2002 May 18;359(9319):1734–9.

67. Fisher B, Anderson S, Bryant J, Margolese RG, Deutsch M, Fisher ER,

et al. Twenty-Year Follow-up of a Randomized Trial Comparing Total Mastectomy, Lumpectomy, and Lumpectomy plus Irradiation for the Treatment of Invasive Breast Cancer. New England Journal of Medicine. 2002 Oct 17;347(16):1233–41.

68. Fiebach J.B., Schellinger P.D., Jansen O., Meyer M., Wilde P., Bender J., et al. CT and Diffusion-Weighted MR Imaging in Randomized Order. Stroke. 2002 Sep 1;33(9):2206–10.

69. Stiell IG, Wells GA, Vandemheen K, Clement C, Lesiuk H, Laupacis A, et al. The Canadian CT Head Rule for patients with minor head injury. The Lancet. 2001 May 5;357(9266):1391–6.

70. Kamath PS, Wiesner RH, Malinchoc M, Kremers W, Therneau TM, Kosberg CL, et al. A model to predict survival in patients with end-stage liver disease. Hepatology. 2001 Feb 1;33(2):464–70.

71. Morris J, Spencer JA, Ambrose NS. MR Imaging Classification of Perianal Fistulas and Its Implications for Patient Management. RadioGraphics. 2000 May 1;20(3):623–35.

72. Mari G, Deter RL, Carpenter RL, Rahman F, Zimmerman R, Moise KJ, et al. Noninvasive Diagnosis by Doppler Ultrasonography of Fetal Anemia Due to Maternal Red-Cell Alloimmunization. New England Journal of Medicine. 2000 Jan 6;342(1):9–14.

73. Acute Respiratory Distress Syndrome Network, Brower RG, Matthay MA, Morris A, Schoenfeld D, Thompson BT, et al. Ventilation with lower tidal volumes as compared with traditional tidal volumes for acute lung injury and the acute respiratory distress syndrome. N Engl J Med. 2000 04;342(18):1301–8.

74. Lee Thomas H., Marcantonio Edward R., Mangione Carol M., Thomas Eric J., Polanczyk Carisi A., Cook E. Francis, et al. Derivation and Prospective Validation of a Simple Index for Prediction of Cardiac Risk of Major Noncardiac Surgery. Circulation. 1999 Sep 7;100(10):1043–9.

75. Kocher MS, Zurakowski D, Kasser JR. Differentiating between septic arthritis and transient synovitis of the hip in children: an evidence-based clinical prediction algorithm. J Bone Joint Surg Am. 1999 Dec;81(12):1662–70.

76. Goodwin SC, McLucas B, Lee M, Chen G, Perrella R, Vedantham S, et al. Uterine Artery Embolization for the Treatment of Uterine Leiomyomata Midterm Results. Journal of Vascular and Interventional Radiology. 1999 Oct 1;10(9):1159–65.

77. Smith-Bindman R, Kerlikowske K, Feldstein VA, Subak L, Scheidler J, Segal M, et al. Endovaginal Ultrasound to Exclude Endometrial Cancer and Other Endometrial Abnormalities. JAMA. 1998 Nov 4;280(17):1510–7.

78. Liberman L, Abramson AF, Squires FB, Glassman JR, Morris EA, Dershaw DD. The breast imaging reporting and data system: positive predictive value of mammographic features and final assessment

categories. American Journal of Roentgenology. 1998 Jul 1;171(1):35–40.

79. Korobkin M, Brodeur FJ, Francis IR, Quint LE, Dunnick NR, Londy F. CT time-attenuation washout curves of adrenal adenomas and nonadenomas. American Journal of Roentgenology. 1998 Mar 1;170(3):747–52.

80. Decousus H, Leizorovicz A, Parent F, Page Y, Tardy B, Girard P, et al. A Clinical Trial of Vena Caval Filters in the Prevention of Pulmonary Embolism in Patients with Proximal Deep-Vein Thrombosis. New England Journal of Medicine. 1998 Feb 12;338(7):409–16.

81. von Kummer R, Allen KL, Holle R, Bozzao L, Bastianello S, Manelfe C, et al. Acute stroke: usefulness of early CT findings before thrombolytic therapy. Radiology. 1997 Nov 1;205(2):327–33.

82. Smith RC, Verga M, McCarthy S, Rosenfield AT. Diagnosis of acute flank pain: value of unenhanced helical CT. American Journal of Roentgenology. 1996 Jan 1;166(1):97–101.

83. Mazzaferro V, Regalia E, Doci R, Andreola S, Pulvirenti A, Bozzetti F, et al. Liver Transplantation for the Treatment of Small Hepatocellular Carcinomas in Patients with Cirrhosis. New England Journal of Medicine. 1996 Mar 14;334(11):693–700.

84. Li H, Boiselle PM, Shepard JO, Trotman-Dickenson B, McLoud TC. Diagnostic accuracy and safety of CT-guided percutaneous needle aspiration biopsy of the lung: comparison of small and large pulmonary nodules. American Journal of Roentgenology. 1996 Jul 1;167(1):105–9.

85. Baron RL, Oliver JH, Dodd GD, Nalesnik M, Holbert BL, Carr B. Hepatocellular carcinoma: evaluation with biphasic, contrast-enhanced, helical CT. Radiology. 1996 May 1;199(2):505–11.

86. van der Wee N, Rinkel GJ, Hasan D, van Gijn J. Detection of subarachnoid haemorrhage on early CT: is lumbar puncture still needed after a negative scan? J Neurol Neurosurg Psychiatry. 1995 Mar;58(3):357–9.

87. Stiell I, Wells G, Laupacis A, Brison R, Verbeek R, Vandemheen K, et al. Multicentre trial to introduce the Ottawa ankle rules for use of radiography in acute ankle injuries. Multicentre Ankle Rule Study Group. BMJ. 1995 Sep 2;311(7005):594–7.

88. Stavros AT, Thickman D, Rapp CL, Dennis MA, Parker SH, Sisney GA. Solid breast nodules: use of sonography to distinguish between benign and malignant lesions. Radiology. 1995 Jul 1;196(1):123–34.

89. National Institute of Neurological Disorders and Stroke rt-PA Stroke Study Group. Tissue plasminogen activator for acute ischemic stroke. N Engl J Med. 1995 14;333(24):1581–7.

90. Korobkin M, Lombardi TJ, Aisen AM, Francis IR, Quint LE, Dunnick NR, et al. Characterization of adrenal masses with chemical shift and

gadolinium-enhanced MR imaging. Radiology. 1995 Nov 1;197(2):411–8.

91. Guibaud L, Bret PM, Reinhold C, Atri M, Barkun AN. Bile duct obstruction and choledocholithiasis: diagnosis with MR cholangiography. Radiology. 1995 Oct 1;197(1):109–15.

92. Rossle M, Haag K, Ochs A, Sellinger M, Noldge G, Perarnau J-M, et al. The Transjugular Intrahepatic Portosystemic Stent-Shunt Procedure for Variceal Bleeding. New England Journal of Medicine. 1994 Jan 20;330(3):165–71.

93. Jensen MC, Brant-Zawadzki MN, Obuchowski N, Modic MT, Malkasian D, Ross JS. Magnetic Resonance Imaging of the Lumbar Spine in People without Back Pain. New England Journal of Medicine. 1994 Jul 14;331(2):69–73.

94. Brown DL, Doubilet PM. Transvaginal sonography for diagnosing ectopic pregnancy: positivity criteria and performance characteristics. Journal of Ultrasound in Medicine. 1994 Apr 1;13(4):259–66.

95. McLoud TC, Bourgouin PM, Greenberg RW, Kosiuk JP, Templeton PA, Shepard JA, et al. Bronchogenic carcinoma: analysis of staging in the mediastinum with CT by correlative lymph node mapping and sampling. Radiology. 1992 Feb 1;182(2):319–23.

96. Lai ECS, Mok FPT, Tan ESY, Lo C, Fan S, You K, et al. Endoscopic Biliary Drainage for Severe Acute Cholangitis. New England Journal of Medicine. 1992 Jun 11;326(24):1582–6.

97. North American Symptomatic Carotid Endarterectomy Trial Collaborators, Barnett HJM, Taylor DW, Haynes RB, Sackett DL, Peerless SJ, et al. Beneficial effect of carotid endarterectomy in symptomatic patients with high-grade carotid stenosis. N Engl J Med. 1991 15;325(7):445–53.

98. Katayama H, Yamaguchi K, Kozuka T, Takashima T, Seez P, Matsuura K. Adverse reactions to ionic and nonionic contrast media. A report from the Japanese Committee on the Safety of Contrast Media. Radiology. 1990 Jun 1;175(3):621–8.

99. Balthazar EJ, Robinson DL, Megibow AJ, Ranson JH. Acute pancreatitis: value of CT in establishing prognosis. Radiology. 1990 Feb 1;174(2):331–6.

100. Lensing AWA, Prandoni P, Brandjes D, Huisman PM, Vigo M, Tomasella G, et al. Detection of Deep-Vein Thrombosis by Real-Time B-Mode Ultrasonography. New England Journal of Medicine. 1989 Feb 9;320(6):342–5.

101. Lensing AWA, Prandoni P, Brandjes D, Huisman PM, Vigo M, Tomasella G, et al. Detection of Deep-Vein Thrombosis by Real-Time B-Mode Ultrasonography. New England Journal of Medicine. 1989 Feb 9;320(6):342–5.

102. Puylaert JBCM, Rutgers PH, Lalisang RI, de Vries BC, van der Werf SDJ, Dörr JPJ, et al. A Prospective Study of Ultrasonography in the Diagnosis of Appendicitis. New

England Journal of Medicine. 1987 Sep 10;317(11):666–9.

103. Bosniak MA. The current radiological approach to renal cysts. Radiology. 1986 Jan 1;158(1):1–10.

104. Harvey RF, Bradshaw JM. A SIMPLE INDEX OF CROHN'S-DISEASE ACTIVITY. The Lancet. 1980 Mar 8;315(8167):514.

105. Fujiwara T, Chida S, Watabe Y, Maeta H, Morita T, Abe T. ARTIFICIAL SURFACTANT THERAPY IN HYALINE-MEMBRANE DISEASE. The Lancet. 1980 Jan 12;315(8159):55–9.

106. Parks AG, Gordon PH, Hardcastle JD. A classification of fistula-in-ano. Br J Surg. 1976 Jan;63(1):1–12.

107. Pugh RN, Murray-Lyon IM, Dawson JL, Pietroni MC, Williams R. Transection of the oesophagus for bleeding oesophageal varices. Br J Surg. 1973 Aug;60(8):646–9.

108. Douglas GJ, Simpson JS. The conservative management of splenic trauma. Journal of Pediatric Surgery. 1971 Oct 1;6(5):565–70.

109. Avery ME, Mead J. Surface Properties in Relation to Atelectasis and Hyaline Membrane Disease. AMA Am J Dis Child. 1959 May 1;97(5_PART_I):517–23.

Statistics Abbreviations

ARI: Absolute Risk Increase
AUC: Area Under the Curve
CI: Confidence Interval
HR: Hazard Ratio
LR: Likelihood Ratio
NNH: Number Needed to Harm
RR: Relative Risk
RRR: Relative Risk Reduction
UL: Uncertainty Limit
X^2: Chi-square

Notes

"The most exciting phrase to hear in science, the one that heralds the most discoveries, is not 'Eureka!', but 'That's funny…' "

- Isaac Asimov, PhD

Made in United States
North Haven, CT
04 November 2026

21760255R00163